Building a United Front: The Critical Role of Global Health Diplomacy

Shiva

Table of Contents

Chapter One: Introduction

Problem Statement

The rapid spread of COVID-19 to every part of the world underscored the need for a swift and coordinated response to current and emerging health threats. Global Health Diplomacy (GHD) was a critical tool in navigating the complexities and interconnectedness of the pandemic and provided the mechanism for a coordinated global response and to secure equitable access to limited health resources. However, the pandemic exposed significant gaps in Global Health Diplomacy actors' knowledge, skills, and competencies, which hindered their ability to effectively respond to a health crisis of this magnitude. Not only is there a critical need to address these gaps as new COVID-19 variants and other infectious diseases emerge, but there is even greater urgency to ensure GHD actors are equipped to effectively navigate and respond to future health challenges.

Explanation

Infectious diseases, pandemics, and bioterrorism threats have been recognized as national and international security threats (Chattu, 2017). With the advancement of globalization, it is becoming more apparent that the resolution of health challenges requires multilevel, multisectoral capabilities, particularly for such issues of global concern and magnitude. The COVID-19 pandemic has underscored countries' increased interconnectedness (Milani, 2020). Global health issues intersect with countries' national interests, competing priorities, power dynamics, and political will. Building consensus among diverse key interest parties (also known as stakeholders) across multiple sectors requires navigating these political factors, aligning interests, and finding common ground through negotiation. This process can be complex, challenging, and time-consuming, considering different countries and organizations have varying agendas and global health priorities, often resulting in conflicting viewpoints (Mac-Seing, Gidey, & Ruggiero, 2023).

Balancing competing needs in resource-limited settings, particularly those characterized by inadequate global health funding, lack of health personnel, and poor health infrastructure, remains challenging (Moyazzem Hossain, Abdulla, & Rahman, 2022). Health behaviors and health outcomes at the individual and population levels are primarily influenced by social, economic, cultural, and historical contexts and disparities that contribute to inequitable healthcare access and poor health. (Khullar & Chokshi, 2018). Therefore, in addition to navigating political dynamics, Global Health Diplomacy actors need to understand the cultural norms, beliefs, and practices surrounding health and health-seeking behaviors, as these directly inform and shape health security priorities and outcomes.

Strengthening Global Health Diplomacy requires GHD actors to have the necessary knowledge, skills, and core competencies to navigate the intersection of public health and foreign policy priorities and build partnerships that foster a collective approach to addressing health threats. These responsibilities require the four Cs of emergency or disaster planning and response: collaboration, communication, coordination, and cooperation (Martin, Nolte, & Vitolo, 2016; Nkengasong, 2023). The four Cs facilitate identifying early warning signs, assessing and mitigating risk, ramping up effective crisis response efforts, and implementing evidence-based strategies. Thus, well-trained Global Health Diplomacy actors are essential for bolstering and sustaining global health security efforts.

Barriers to Global Health Diplomacy

Global Health Diplomacy efforts were tested when the world was faced with a public health pandemic. The GHD response to COVID-19 mitigation efforts demonstrated in real time the need for a cohesive, coordinated global response to address the pandemic. With COVID-19 no longer considered a Public Health Emergency of International Concern, public health leadership is at an opportune moment to engage in strategic planning to understand and tackle the obstacles and barriers that surfaced during the crisis.

Lack of international coordination: The months leading up to and those following the WHO's declaration of COVID-19 as a Public Health Emergency of International Concern revealed the lack of global cooperation and coordination (Jones & Hameiri, 2022). Every country appeared to have varying pandemic preparedness, uncoordinated response levels, and variable approaches to engaging a public health response. These differences resulted in the implementation of isolated prevention and mitigation strategies such as restrictions on trade and travel, stay-at-home orders, social distancing measures, and mask mandates (Sirleaf & Clark, 2021). The lack of coordination hampered efforts to manage the crisis effectively.

Political tensions and conflicts: The existing rivalry and political tensions between nations hindered real-time information and resource sharing (Dhami et al., 2022). These factors are critical to Global Health Diplomacy practice and promoting a collective pandemic response and a joint response to any other global health emergency. COVID-19 also increased political and social unrest within countries, compounded by pandemic fatigue that stemmed from prolonged and changing restrictions of varying severity (Jørgensen et al., 2022).

Vaccine equity and access: The pandemic underscored stark inequities in the availability, affordability, and access to vaccines that persist to this day. The disparities in equitable vaccine distribution amongst countries, particularly between high-income and low- and middle-income countries (LMICs), manifested as vaccine nationalism. Vaccine nationalism is "an economic strategy to hoard vaccinations from manufacturers and increase supply in their own country" (Riaz et al., 2021). In the race to manufacture and purchase COVID-19 vaccines, many developed countries prioritized the needs of their citizens through a 'my country first' or 'every nation for itself' approach over global solidarity, putting more people at risk (Guterres, 2021). The health and well-being of people from LMICs who lacked the technology, expertise, and ability to develop their own vaccines were similarly neglected in the COVID-19 vaccine response. Wealthier countries' decisions to roll out COVID-19 boosters, while many low-income countries were yet to secure the first round of single-dose vaccines, sparked significant controversy. Research data from 152 countries estimates that over a million lives may have been lost in LMICs due to wealthier nations hoarding COVID-19 vaccines (Ledford, 2022).

Disinformation and misinformation: The spread of disinformation and misinformation during the pandemic is arguably one of the most significant obstacles to Global Health Diplomacy (Tagliabue, Galassi, & Mariani, 2020). Uncertainties about the virus's nature, effects, virulence, and allegations about its origins served as fodder for false information, undermining trust among nations. Mis-and-disinformation campaigns, rumors, and conspiracy theories eroded the public's trust in public health authorities and global health institutions (Lewandowsky, Linden, & Norman, 2024), making implementing effective public health measures difficult. The speed at which the COVID-19 vaccines were developed also contributed to global vaccine skepticism and hesitancy, expressed as people's reluctance or unwillingness to get vaccinated (Wiysonge et al., 2021). These factors resulted in a lack of cooperation among countries and reluctance to share accurate data, making coordinating the international response even more challenging.

Economic constraints: Insufficient funding for pandemic prevention, preparedness, and response remains a global challenge despite the recent history of epidemics and infectious disease outbreaks. The economic impact of the pandemic also affected Global Health Diplomacy actors' efforts to elicit dedicated funding for the pandemic response. Many countries grappled with the challenge of allocating resources for international assistance while simultaneously addressing the growing demands of their own citizens and the needs of their health systems (Kaye et al., 2021).

Geopolitical rivalries: The pandemic exacerbated existing geopolitical rivalry and power struggles and highlighted significant issues plaguing multilateral systems over the past decade. The geopolitical impasse and heightened tensions in diplomatic relations between the United States and China were particularly glaring, underscored by the lack of trust and information sharing about the origin of the virus (Zhou, 2024). This standoff forestalled the advancement of the multilateral discussions and pandemic response efforts at the WHO and the U.N. Security Council. As the pandemic progressed, China strove to assert its dominance (Chen, Rodewald, Lai, & Gao, 2021) and geographic influence through its stringent initial and sustained containment measures (Ding & Zhang, 2022). The United States, under the Trump administration, on the other hand, faced immense criticism about the delays in its pandemic response, as well as contradictory COVID-19 messaging and preventative measures. The geopolitical rivalry impeded international cooperation as countries like Japan questioned the WHO's deference to China's political calculations, with its deputy Prime Minister dubbing the WHO the "Chinese Health Organization" (Fidler, 2020). Former President Trump also called out the WHO for "becoming too China-centric," which in part led to his decision to freeze US contributions to the WHO and his announcement of the American Government's intention to withdraw its WHO membership. The ongoing rivalry overshadowed the urgency and need for international cooperation to effectively address the pandemic.

Limited resources and capacity in LMICS: A significant concern among low-and-middle-income countries (LMICs) was their ability to control the spread of the virus while managing the high infectious disease burden within their health systems. These countries' limited financial, infrastructural, and human resources, particularly those in the sub-Saharan African region, hampered their pandemic response capacity (Haldane et al., 2021). The pandemic caused disruptions to health systems supply chains as travel restrictions affected the transportation and delivery of essential health equipment and supplies and the movement of essential health personnel and GHD actors (Boro & Stoll, 2022). These disruptions contributed to health facilities and the public not having access to personal protective equipment, water, sanitation, and hygiene facilities, a lack of vaccines, diagnostic tests, and medical supplies, and the inability to access healthcare services. These disparities also hindered these countries' active participation or leverage in Global Health Diplomacy discussions around knowledge-sharing and resource allocation (Bayati, Noroozi, Ghanbari-Jahromi, & Jalali, 2022).

Key Definitions

Global Health, as defined by the World Health Organization, is "an area for study, research, and practice that places a priority on improving health and achieving health equity for all people worldwide" (Koplan et al., 2009).

Global health diplomacy is "an interdisciplinary field that bridges global public health, international relations, and multisectoral public policy with a goal to achieve global health" (Kickbusch et al., 2021). This description accentuates the World Health Organization's multistakeholder approach to GHD to 1) Improve health security and population health; 2) Revamp interstate relationships and their commitment to working collaboratively to improve health; and 3) Alleviate poverty and foster equity through fair and just outcomes (WHO, n.d.).

Global Health Security (also Health Security) is the "existence of strong and resilient public health systems that can prevent, detect, and respond to infectious disease threats, wherever they occur in the world" (CDC.gov, 2023).

Within this study, the researcher uses the terms "Global Health Diplomacy actors" or "actors" for short to mean individuals, government agencies, institutions, organizations, or entities that cultivate interactions and negotiations between and among each other and within and across governments and states, with the principal objective of improving population health.

Purpose of the Study

This exploratory, descriptive qualitative study seeks to investigate the knowledge, skills, and competencies required by GHD actors to effectively practice Global Health Diplomacy. The study will be underpinned by a Grounded Theory approach, which will allow the researcher to "see" the research problem through the "eyes" of GHD practitioners. This approach will also facilitate the presentation of more targeted solutions grounded in the data that emerged from the interviewees' perspectives (Glaser & Strauss, 2017) on the knowledge, skills, and core competencies required for GHD practice in a post-COVID era. Although the study will focus on the US GHD actors, the interdependence of Global Health Diplomacy may allow the study results to be utilized in different countries and contexts as a bridge between scholarship and practice.

This research builds upon key findings by Katz et al., 2011. In their study *"Defining Health Diplomacy: Changing Demands in the Era of Globalization,"* they proposed a taxonomy for classifying Global Health Diplomacy (GHD) actors into three distinct categories: Core, Multistakeholder, and Informal (Katz et al., 2011). This study called for a reassessment of the necessary skills, understanding, and resources for each group to achieve their collective goals. Brown et al., 2018 sought to bridge the gap between foreign policy and public health objectives by examining the multidisciplinary role of Health Attachés in diplomacy and statecraft. Their study called for standardized training for Core GHD actors and professionalization of the field of Global Health Diplomacy. In addition, their study proposed a Global Health Diplomacy Pyramid using defining constructs advanced by Katz et al. in 2011 (see Figure 1).

The Global Health Diplomacy Pyramid depicts the actors and tools within each of the three main GHD categories (Brown et al., 2014). The number of actors increases as one moves from the Health Attachés and diplomats at the Core at the apex of the pyramid to the representatives in the informal sector at the base. There is a corresponding decrease in role specificity from the Core to the Informal Health Diplomacy actors. However, this pyramid does not reflect the effectiveness of one category over another, as each group of actors is equally relevant and plays a central role in Global Health Diplomacy negotiations and the development of global health strategies or foreign policy goals in different contexts. While certain Global Health Diplomacy tools have been ascribed to specific categories, their use is not necessarily restricted to these groups.

Figure 1
Pyramid of Global Health Diplomacy

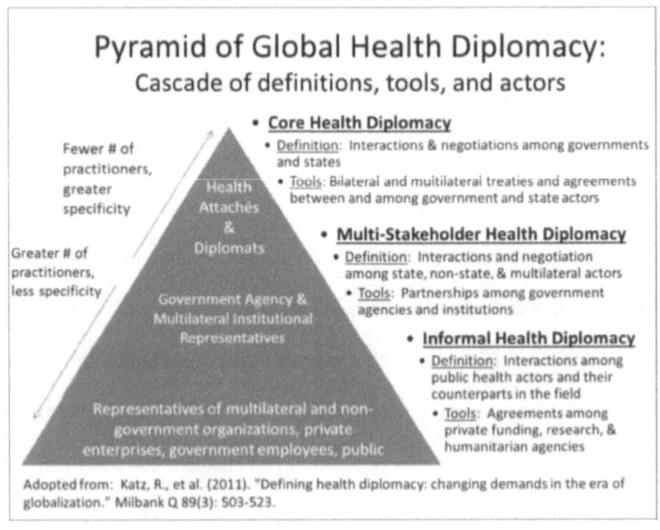

(Brown et al., 2018)

Study Aims and Research Questions

This study seeks to achieve the following aims:

Aim 1: Determine the required skills and core competencies for Global Health Diplomacy practice for each GHD actor role.

The researcher defines "skills" as specific learned abilities required to successfully practice Global Health Diplomacy. The researcher defines "core competencies" as the essential knowledge, skills, and abilities that GHD actors need to effectively practice Global Health Diplomacy and the proper application of these knowledge, skills, and abilities at the right place and time. The researcher defines "Global Health Diplomacy Actors" as individuals, government agencies, institutions, organizations, or entities that cultivate interactions and negotiations between and among each other and within and across governments and states, with the principal objective of improving population health.

Research Question 1: What skills do GHD actors need for effective Global Health Diplomacy practice in a post-COVID era?

Research Question 2: What core competencies do GHD actors need for effective Global Health Diplomacy practice in a post-COVID era?

Aim 2: Identify technical knowledge gaps for each Global Health Diplomacy actor category.

The researcher defines "technical knowledge" as the practical or theoretical understanding of Global Health Diplomacy.

Research Question 3: What technical knowledge gaps exist amongst Global Health

Diplomacy actors?

Aim 3: Define Global Health Diplomacy in a post-COVID era.

"Define," as used by the researcher, means to describe or explain the meaning of

Global Health Diplomacy based on the GHD actor's understanding of knowledge, skills,

and competencies required for practice in a post-COVID era.

Research Question 4: How do Global Health Diplomacy actors define Global Health

Diplomacy in a post-COVID era?

Aim 4: Generate a summary of core competency requirements for GHD practice in a

post-COVID era based on data from each GHD actor level.

The researcher anticipates that this information will be used to inform the

development of targeted training for each category of GHD actors.

Study Rationale

The pandemic underscored the need to strengthen global health security and

preparedness, increase equitable access to COVID-19 vaccines, diagnostics, and

treatment, combat vaccine hesitancy, strengthen health systems, foster health equity,

address health inequalities, and build economic resilience. These priorities required

bilateral and multilateral diplomatic engagement at the national and subnational level for

a collaborative approach that promotes ownership, trust, transparency, accountability, and

timely evidence-informed decision-making for a strong and targeted pandemic response.

Within the United States, Global health Diplomacy has been recognized as a

critical foreign policy tool and a pivotal contributor to national security. The COVID-19 pandemic accentuated the United States' crucial role in global health and health security

(Blinken, 2023). Different Global Health Diplomacy goals will employ a variety of actors

whose roles and duties may evolve within the scope and context of specific objectives.

For example, while the responsibility of Global Health Diplomacy negotiations and

policymaking within the US may rest with the State and its institutions, the role of

healthcare providers, public health professionals, and researchers in program and policy

design cannot be overlooked (Katz et al., 2011). Similarly, ongoing negotiations such as

the amendments to the International Health Regulations and the Pandemic Agreement

require sharing these responsibilities with other international organizations such as the

U.N., WHO, foreign affairs ministers, ambassadors, health attaches, or other GHD actors

(WHO.int, 2023).

The overarching goal of diplomatic negotiations during the pandemic was to

promote collective action to mitigate the effects of COVID-19, shore up equitable access

to vaccines, diagnostics, and treatment, save lives, and leverage foreign policy to end the

pandemic as quickly as possible. Some of these negotiations by GHD actors resulted in

securing agreements for manufacturing and distributing COVID-19 vaccines and

designated funding for procuring critical resources, including medical equipment and

supplies. The earlier months of the pandemic saw a marked global increase in the demand

for diagnostic tests, PPE, masks, ventilators, etc., amid global supply shortages.

Furthermore, GHD actors facilitated the development of policy guidelines for

preventive public health measures, domestic and international travel, and trade

restrictions to minimize the spread of the virus. They also brokered innovative public-private partnerships, fostered data and scientific information sharing, secured aid for vulnerable populations, and funding for health systems strengthening.

Research Imperative

Global Health Diplomacy is central to facilitating and assuring global prevention, preparedness, and response efforts to imminent health threats with immediacy and intentionality (Blinken, 2023). Research predicts a 38% percent likelihood that another pandemic as severe as COVID-19 will occur during our lifetimes due to risk factors from globalization, climate change, and human conflict (Marani, Katul, Pan, & Parolari, 2021). The question of where the next global health threat will emerge looms as COVID-19 lessens in intensity (USAID.gov, 2023). Lowering the chances of another global health threat from occurring will require significant diplomacy efforts through a whole-of-government and a whole-of-society approach to strengthen early detection, global pandemic preparedness, and coordinated response (State.gov., 2021).

The Global Health Diplomat serves as the front-line practitioner for GHD. However, the role of the Diplomat cannot remain static and must, like our public health efforts, change and respond. Global Health Diplomacy objectives can be grouped into two categories: health for diplomacy and diplomacy for health. Health for diplomacy strategically utilizes health-related policies, initiatives, or interventions to advance diplomatic goals and achieve positive diplomatic outcomes. Diplomacy for health leverages bilateral and multilateral diplomatic efforts and interactions to respond to global health threats, achieve global health objectives, and address health challenges for positive health outcomes.

The revision of the role requires identifying the knowledge, skills, and core competencies for practicing Global Health Diplomacy in a post-COVID era (State.gov., 2023). This research will draw from critical lessons learned from the recent pandemic and how these can inform the training and development of present-day and future Global Health Diplomacy actors to deliver on their mission of preventing, preparing for, and responding to current and future health security threats.

According to Kickbusch et al., 2021 "ensuring that diplomats have a combination of different skills increases the professionalism of global health diplomacy negotiations and the likelihood of achieving successful outcomes." Developing these skills builds the capacity of current and future GHD professionals, and practicing them in real-life scenarios like the World Health Assembly (WHA) is increasingly being recognized as a critical component of their training.

Multilateral negotiation scenarios require diplomats and experts from the different member states to perform various formal and informal functions (WHO, 2023). These negotiations may have structured plenary sessions, committee meetings, or other formal functions that include regional consultations or meetings of drafting groups. Global Health Diplomacy actors are also expected to participate in informal discussions with non-state actors or counterparts from countries with similar interests. Informal interactions that may occur during coordination meetings, technical briefings, side events, receptions, and coffee breaks are equally important.

The diversity in background and range of experience of GHD actors can be considered assets to Global Health Diplomacy as these attributes may be leveraged in critical diplomatic interactions. Nevertheless, the growing demands within global health security warrant multidisciplinary skills and multisectoral coordination, particularly amongst Core GHD actors whose roles often require greater specificity and designated outcomes.

This study will employ a Grounded Theory descriptive qualitative design using semi-structured in-depth interviews to explore the knowledge, skills, and core competencies that GHD actors require for effective Global Health Diplomacy practice in a post-COVID era.

Chapter Two: Literature Review

This chapter presents a literature review on the research topic *Defining Global Health Diplomacy in a post-COVID Era: Investigating the knowledge, skills, and core competencies required by GHD actors to address current and future global health threats.* A literature review surveys credible information sources on a topic, selects relevant and timely research information, and summarizes, synthesizes, and critiques this information in writing (Leite, Padilha, & Cecatti, 2019). This work appraises the evolution of GHD, its relevance and timeliness, challenges faced by GHD actors, the role of the United States and its actors in this field, professionalization of the field, and implications for practice in a post-COVID era. The review combines grey literature and published journal articles.

Literature Review Methodology

The Researcher carried out a literature search for scholarly publications between October 7 and October 17, 2023, using four electronic databases: The George Washington University Himmelfarb Library Articles + GW & Consortium, the George Washington University Gelman Articles + GW & Consortium Catalog, PUBMED, and Google Scholar for journal articles on Global Health Diplomacy in a post-COVID era. This search focused on journal articles published between 2019 and 2023 in English. Journal articles that did not meet the inclusion criteria were excluded from the review.

The search terms included "Global Health Diplomacy knowledge skills competencies in a post-COVID Era" and produced 10,200 results. The search phrase was used in conjunction with "Global Health Security" and "gaps," as well as with alternative terms for "skills and competencies," such as "expertise" or "techniques," to ensure articles were aligned with the research's aims. These additional terms further distilled the search results to 155, including 53 journal articles. Search results were not restricted by geography to ensure pertinent publications were not missed.

A similar search was run through the George Washington University Himmelfarb Library Articles + GW & Consortium and the George Washington University Gelman Articles + GW & Consortium Catalog databases; however, the results were not as comprehensive as those from Google Scholar. Upon verification, the Researcher found that some articles from these databases were also included in the Google Scholar search, and duplicates were eliminated.

The abstracts of 53 journal articles were read for relevance to the research aims, and 34 more that were not relevant to the research topic were excluded. In total, the researcher retained 19 peer-reviewed journal articles that specifically addressed either knowledge, skills, or competencies of Global Health Diplomacy in line with current and future global health security threats and priorities. The search did not yield any journal articles that addressed all three study domains (knowledge, skills, and core competencies). Key articles are summarized in Table 5, and the remaining articles and grey literature have been integrated into the narrative review below.

The History and Evolution of Global Health Diplomacy

Over the years, the field of Global Health Diplomacy has evolved, predominantly driven by the fluctuating nature of health security threats (Novotny, 2013). Although global "microbial unification" began around 1492 through the cross-country and cross-continental spread of epidemics, mainly between Europe and Asia, it took over 300 years

for countries to recognize the shared risk of disease pathogens (Berlinguer, 1999). These

changes emerged with a noticeable shift in the understanding of human security from the

need to protect one's personal environment and prolong territorial integrity to a broader

concern for humanity's well-being (Novotny, 2013). Globalization has been a critical

factor in cross-border infectious disease control and the need for international health

cooperation that has shaped diplomatic relations between countries over the past 160

years (Kickbusch & Ivanova, 2013).

The term 'globalization' was first coined by Theodore Levitt in 1983 following

the Industrial Revolution (Volle, 2023). However, some scholars date it back to 1870,

employing the term to mean "interconnection, intensification,

and accelerating interdependence" or, according to social scientists, "the stretching of

economic, political, and social relationships in space and time" (Volle, 2023). Between

500 BC and 1700 AD, public health history records these interconnections that

demonstrate how events in one part of the world affected the health of populations in

others (Tulchinsky & Varavikova, 2014). However, it was not until the mid-19th century

that states began cooperating internationally to mitigate the risks to human health

worldwide, mainly by developing, deploying, and administering vaccines (Hotez, 2014).

In addition to addressing infectious diseases, GHD has provided opportunities for

negotiation, collective action by policymakers, and national and international

multistakeholder engagements to stem morbidity and mortality resulting from non-

communicable diseases and to strengthen existing health systems (Asadi-Lari et al.,

2021).

Fidler provided an analysis of international health diplomacy, spanning the mid-18th – mid-19th century, shedding light on how lessons from the past may influence current and future states of global health governance (Fidler, 2001). In commemoration of its 75th Anniversary, the World Health Organization highlighted several critical public health milestones from its inception in 1945 (WHO.int, 2023). These events from 1851 to the present day have defined the history and evolution of Global Health Diplomacy, some of which are highlighted below.

1851: Beginning of International Health Diplomacy; European States gathered for the first International Sanitary Conference to discuss collaboration on the Plague, Yellow Fever, and Cholera (WHO.int, 2023).

1902: The Pan American Health Organization was established by 11 North, South, and Latin American countries to protect population health and regional economic stability by preventing the spread of epidemics between countries. In 1903, the US signed the Hay-Herrán Treaty, securing authorization to build the Panama Canal (PAHO, n.d.).

1924: The League of Nations, the first-ever intergovernmental organization, was created at the end of World War I to foster multilateral cooperation and promote peace and security amongst nations (UNGeneva.org. n.d.). The organization was dissolved 26 years later due to its inability to enforce its decisions effectively and deter military aggression and conflict (History.State.gov, n.d.).

April 1945: Diplomats met at the UN Conference in San Francisco, California. Brazil and Chinese Diplomats underscored the need for better global collaboration and organization to address global health threats, calling for the creation of the World Health Organization (WHO.int, 2023).

1946: The WHO constitution was proposed, drafted, and adopted at the International Health Conference in New York, with 61 signatories: 51 UN member state representatives and ten from other countries (WHO.int, 2023).

1947: The World Health Organization set up the first-ever global disease tracking service (WHO.int, 2023).

April 7, 1948: The World Health Organization constitution came into full effect. The date was commemorated after that as World Health Day (WHO.int, 2023).

1955: The WHO launched a program to eradicate malaria globally. Malaria had already been eliminated in the US 4 years earlier (CDC.gov, 2022).

1967: The WHO relaunched the Intensified Smallpox Eradication Program after initial efforts two years prior yielded unsatisfactory results (WHO.int, 2023).

1969: The WHO Member States adopted the first set of International Health Regulations at the World Health Assembly. This agreement called for cooperation and collaboration amongst member states to prevent and respond to public health threats of transnational potential (WHO.int, 2023).

1978: The WHO established the ambitious "Health for All" goal at the Alma-Ata International Conference on Primary Healthcare in Kazakhstan, setting the stage for calls for Universal Health Coverage (WHO.int, 2023).

1980: The WHO announced the elimination of smallpox at the thirty-third World Health Assembly, following a 12-year intensive vaccination campaign (WHO.int, 2023).

1981: WHO Member States adopted the International Code of Marketing Breastmilk Substitutes to address marketing, advertising, and education efforts to dissuade mothers from breastfeeding. By 2022, some legal stipulations of the Code had been enforced by three-quarters of countries, resulting in a 50% increase in exclusive breastfeeding rates (WHO.int, 2023).

1983: The human immunodeficiency virus (HIV) was discovered. The virus went on to cause the AIDS pandemic (WHO.int, 2023).

1988: The WHO Member States launched the Global Polio Eradication Initiative (GPEI) at the World Health Assembly when the disease was endemic in 125 countries. In 2022, WHO announced that polio had been eliminated in all but two countries worldwide (WHO.int, 2023).

1999: GAVI (formerly the Global Alliance for Vaccines and Immunization) was established. The Alliance constituted the WHO, UN agencies, prominent foundations and actors in the vaccine development industry, and government officials to increase childhood vaccine availability and access (WHO.int, 2023).

1999: The WHO established the first-ever global strategy to prevent and control non-communicable diseases (WHO.int, 2023).

2000: The United Nations Millenium Declaration was adopted in the largest-ever gathering of world leaders. The declaration elicited global partnership and commitment towards eight Millennium Development Goals for the next 15 years. Several of these had health as a specific target, as well as alleviating extreme poverty, reducing hunger, and combatting illiteracy, discrimination against women, and environmental degradation (WHO.int, 2023).

2000: The WHO established the Global Outbreak Alert and Response Network (GOARN) to detect and fight the spread of outbreaks from one country to another (WHO.int, 2023).

2001: The UN General Assembly announced a Declaration of Commitment on HIV/AIDS to support and encourage comprehensive, multilevel coordination and collaboration to fight the spread of the disease (WHO.int, 2023).

2001: The Global Fund to Fight AIDS, Tuberculosis, and Malaria was created in partnership with UN agencies, WHO, and major donors (WHO.int, 2023).

2002: The African Union was launched, replacing the Organization of African Unity (OAU). Its mission is to foster unity and solidarity on the continent through cooperation, safeguard national sovereignty, and represent the interests and well-being of Africans within intergovernmental organizations (AU.int., n.d.).

February 2003: The WHO announced a severe acute respiratory syndrome (SARS) outbreak, a viral respiratory infection that appeared in China and spread to four other countries (Mackenzie, n.d.). The WHO activated the Global Outbreak Alert and Response Network to rapidly identify and deploy volunteers while disseminating public health measures to control the spread (WHO.int, 2023).

2003: The President's Emergency Plan for AIDS Relief (PEPFAR) was created, showcasing the US Government's commitment to eliminating HIV/AIDS (State.gov, 2023).

2003: The Framework Convention on Tobacco Control was unanimously adopted by the World Health Assembly as WHO's first-ever global public health treaty to reduce tobacco-related morbidity and mortality (WHO.int, 2023).

2005: The International Health Regulations were revised to provide states with more explicit guidelines for reporting public health emergencies and disease outbreaks to the WHO and isolation and containment protocols (WHO.int, 2023).

2005: The European Centers for Disease Control was established as the European Union public health agency with the goal of providing regional guidance and support to countries on prevention and response to public health threats and infectious disease outbreaks (ECDC, 2017).

2009: A new H1N1 influenza virus, also known as the swine flu, was thought to have emerged in Mexico, causing the WHO to declare its first-ever Public Health Emergency of International Concern (PHEIC) (WHO.int, 2023). A PHEIC is "an extraordinary event which is determined to constitute a public health risk to other States through the international spread of disease and to potentially require a coordinated international response" (WHO.int, 2019). The WHO's collaboration with pharmaceutical companies facilitated the development of a new influenza vaccine in record time (WHO.int, 2023).

2011: The Pandemic Influenza Preparedness (PIP) Framework developed by WHO Member States was unanimously adopted at the 64th World Health Assembly (WHO.int, 2023). The PIP Framework was designed to bring together leaders, governments, and diverse stakeholders to promote equitable access and availability of vaccines and pandemic-related supplies and foster the sharing of influenza viruses with the potential to cause human pandemics (WHO.int, 2022).

2011: The Caribbean Public Health Agency (CARPHA) was created by the Caribbean Community (CARICOM countries) as the public health agency for the Caribbean region, with the goal of promoting regional solidarity and preventing and responding to emergencies in member states (CARPHA, 2022).

2014: The Ebola outbreak emerged in Guinea and rapidly spread to neighboring Liberia and Sierra Leone and then to seven other countries, including the United States, United Kingdom, Spain, Senegal, Nigeria, Mali, and Italy, prompting the WHO to declare a PHEIC (WHO.int, 2023). In response to the outbreak, the WHO secretariat mobilized foreign medical teams, deployed technical experts, support staff, and equipment, and set up mobile treatment centers and laboratories (WHO.int, 2023).

2014: The Director-General of WHO declared a Public Health Emergency of International Concern (PHEIC) due to its spread across nine countries, with accompanying recommendations for vaccinations for international travelers (WHO.int., 2014).

2015: The 2030 Agenda for 17 Sustainable Development Goals was adopted by UN Member States. These goals comprised 169 wide-ranging and interconnecting targets; amongst them Goal 3, which aims to "ensure healthy lives and promote well-being for all at all ages" (WHO.int, 2023).

2016: The Africa CDC was established by the African Union's 26th Ordinary Assembly of Heads of State and Government to strengthen the continent's efforts in preventing, preparing, and responding to global health threats (Africa CDC, 2019).

2016: The UN Member States adopted a political declaration on Antimicrobial Resistance (AMR) at the UN General Assembly meeting, with calls for interagency coordination efforts to develop practical guidelines to ensure multilateral cooperation to combat AMR (WHO.int, 2023).

2016: The WHO declared Zika a Public Health Emergency of International Concern following a 2015 outbreak in Brazil and proven links to microcephaly and neurological defects in newborns (WHO.int, 2023). So far, evidence of mosquito-borne, Zika-related infections has been registered in 86 countries (WHO.int, 2023).

2019: The UN Political Declaration on Universal Health Coverage was adopted by Member States as a landmark commitment to make primary healthcare more accessible, affordable, and equitable (WHO.int, 2023).

2020: The WHO declared COVID-19 a Public Health Emergency of International Concern (WHO.int, 2023).

2022: The WHO Member States agreed to consider revising specific amendments to the 2005 International Health Regulations based on events surrounding the COVID-19 pandemic (WHO.int, 2023).

2023: The US Secretary of State Antony Blinken launched the Department of State Bureau of Global Health Security and Diplomacy, tasked with coordinating US foreign assistance and fostering multilateral cooperation at the national, regional, and international levels to prevent global health threats (State.gov, 2023).

2023: Global leaders adopted a political declaration on pandemic prevention, preparedness, and response at the United Nations General Assembly to fire up Pandemic Treaty negotiations (UN.org, 2023).

The events mentioned above require diplomatic engagements to adapt yet again, considering growing global health and environmental challenges (Kickbusch & Ivanova, 2013). The role of health diplomats has also evolved to include the dual responsibility of managing countries' interdependence while representing national and communal interests (Sending, Pouliot & Neumann, 2011). Diplomacy among countries remains critical, warranting that bilateral and multilateral partnerships developed over the past 200 years are leveraged to manage ongoing changes to the global health landscape (Mahbubani, 2022). These duties recognized the need for negotiating binding trade and economic agreements within the health and environmental sectors (ITC, 2023). Thus, emerging and existing global health threats, multilevel interactions, the diversity in GHD actors, and changes to the rules, norms, and expectations account for the state of flux of Global Health Diplomacy (Kickbusch & Ivanova, 2013).

Review of Global Health Diplomacy Definitions

Almeida, 2020 reviewed some definitions of the terms "Global Health Diplomacy (GHD)" or "Health Diplomacy (HD)." Existing literature suggests a lack of consensus; "HD and GHD mean different things to different authors, and definitions were coined to address the notion of global health, which appeared around the same time. The terms are often associated with contemporary globalization, but are also in dialogue with yet another, earlier expression: international health" (Almeida, 2020). Amid the differences in definitions of GHD or HD, certain commonalities are highlighted, such as the interdependence between international relations and health, the role of diverse actors, and multilevel negotiations for consensus-building around health efforts. Almeida, 2020 also notes that the "descriptive, functional, or instrumental approach to GHD" underpinning each definition depended on the authors' global perspective and timeline. Table 1 below captures the selected definitions retained by the author that emerged between 2007 and 2017.

Table 1
Global Health Diplomacy Definitions

Definition	Reference
"Health is a catalyst for the rearrangement of powerful interests within government. It sets a new standard against which foreign policy can be measured. Health moves foreign policy away from a debate about national interests to one about global altruism."	Horton (2007, p. 807)
"The term global health diplomacy aims to capture (…) multilevel and multi-actor negotiation processes that shape and manage the global policy environment for health."	Kickbusch, Silberschmidt, and Buss (2007, p. 230)
"[Global health diplomacy is] an emerging field that addresses the dual goals of improving global health and bettering international relations, particularly in conflict areas and in resource-poor environments."	Adams et al. (2008, p. 316)
"[GHD is . . .] the cultivation of trust and negotiation of mutual benefit in the context of global health goals."	Bond (2008, p. 377)
"Health Diplomacy is the chosen method of interaction between stakeholders engaged in public health and politics for the purpose of representation, cooperation, resolving disputes, improving health systems, and securing the right to health for vulnerable populations."	Health Diplomats, cited by Lee and Smith (2011, p. 1)

"Global health is an area for study, research, and practice that places a priority on improving health and achieving equity in health for all people worldwide. Global health emphasizes transnational health issues, determinants, and solutions; involves many disciplines within and beyond the health sciences and promotes interdisciplinary collaboration; and is a synthesis of population-based prevention with individual-level clinical care."	Koplan et al. (2009, p. 1995)
"'Global health diplomacy' refers to both a system of organization and to communication and negotiation processes that shape the global policy environment in the sphere of health and its determinants."	Kickbusch and Kökény (2013, p. 159)
"[A working definition of health diplomacy is] the policy-shaping processes through which States, intergovernmental organizations, and non-State actors negotiate responses to health challenges or utilize health concepts or mechanisms in policy-shaping and negotiation strategies to achieve other political, economic, or social objectives."	Fidler (2013, p. 693)
"GHD refers to international diplomatic activities that (directly or indirectly) address issues of global health importance, and is concerned with how and why global health issues play out in a foreign policy context."	Michaud and Kates (2013, p. 24)
"Global health diplomacy (GHD) has emerged as a concept to describe the practices by which governments and non-state actors attempt to coordinate efforts to improve global health."	Ruckert et al. (2016, p. 61)
"GHD focuses on international negotiation, which includes a range of processes, from finalising agreements between multilateral or bilateral aid donors and recipient countries, to the processes of making binding and non-binding international agreements in health or related to health."	Smith and Irwin (2016, p. 1)
"[GHD] refers both to formal multilateral and bilateral decision-making around health, and to the interaction between health and foreign policy concerns (such as 'health security') involving negotiations and cooperation among a range of state and non-state actors."	Birn, Muntaner, and Afzal (2017, p. S38), based on the findings of various authors, most cited in this table

Adapted from Almeida, 2020

More Recent Global Health Diplomacy Definitions

More recent definitions of Global Health Diplomacy emerged within the same time frame as the COVID-19 pandemic (2019 to present). These newer definitions share some similarities to the previous definitions and encompass the 4 Cs in the mission statement of the new Bureau of Global Health Security and Diplomacy: Coordination, Collaboration, Cooperation, and Communication (Nkengasong, 2023).

"Global health diplomacy focuses on those health issues that need the cooperation of many countries to address issues of common concern, but health diplomacy can also play a central role at the regional, bilateral, and national level" (WHO.int, 2022).

"Global health diplomacy is a sociopolitical practice involving the global health policy community, which promotes the interrelationship between health and foreign policy both at the national level, through cooperation projects or international actions and, in international arenas, by acting in global political space in the widest range of spheres, whether health-sector-related or otherwise" (Almeida, 2020)

"Global health diplomacy is at the intersection of public health and foreign affairs, to foster critical relationships with multilateral organizations, foreign governments, and Ministries of Health and Science and Technology around the world" (OGA 2023).

"Global Health Diplomacy (GHD) is the practice by which governments and non-state actors attempt to coordinate global policy solutions to improve global health" (PAHO, n.d.).

"Global Health Diplomacy is a method of interaction between the different stakeholders of the public health sector in a bid to promote representation, cooperation, promotion of the right to health and improvement of health systems for vulnerable populations on a global scale. It is the link between health and international relations" (Gov.UK, 2021).

The Intersection of Health, Foreign Policy, and Global Health Governance

As demonstrated by the evolution of GHD, while health has been interwoven into countries' foreign policy agendas, it has risen and fallen as a foreign policy priority (Fidler, 2011). Foreign policy refers to the "policies a state advances in relations with other states, intergovernmental organizations (IGOs), and non-state actors (e.g., non-governmental organizations) on issues that have cross-border consequences" (Fidler, 2011). Global health governance is "the use of formal and informal institutions, rules, and processes by states, intergovernmental organizations, and non-state actors to deal with challenges to health that require cross-border collective action to address effectively" (Fidler, 2010). Health diplomacy engagements seek to strengthen global health governance, build relationships, and foster cooperation at national, regional, and international levels to improve foreign policy.

Over the past decades, global health challenges like SARS, Ebola, and HIV/AIDS have risen to become top foreign policy priorities. These issues have warranted increased attention from policymakers and health governance bodies, increased funding to tackle these problems, and expanded scholarship exploring the link between health and foreign policy (IOM, 2009). In 2010, Feldbaum, Lee & Michaud examined the role of health in four foreign policy domains, including aid, diplomacy, trade, and national security. They ascribed countries' inclinations to act on health challenges to their foreign policy interests rather than the desire for more accessible and equitable health care. Some of these interests could be diplomatic (bilateral and multilateral collaboration for epidemic prevention, economic (trade protection), strategic (prevention of bio, nuclear, and cyber terrorism), or oftentimes a combination of these (Feldbaum, Lee & Michaud, 2010).

Health For Diplomacy

Health can be a tool for achieving diplomatic outcomes such as conflict resolution, peace, sustainable development, economic stability, poverty reduction, social justice, and human rights (Cho, 2023). Many of these efforts can be accomplished through negotiations.

Negotiations in Global Health

Negotiation is "a process of exchange between two or more interested parties for the purpose of reaching agreement on issues of mutual concern" (Lister et al., 2012). This process constitutes three main phases: Phase 1, also known as the diagnostic phase, identifies critical issues for negotiation, engages relevant stakeholders, and prepares information to be shared. In phase 2, or the formula phase, an agreement framework and exchange process is established and communicated. The negotiation and exchange process occurs in phase 3, or the detailed phase (Zartman & Berman, 1982).

Negotiating health agreements is crucial to health diplomacy objectives and relies on countries' willingness to communicate, cooperate, and collaborate (Odell & Tingley, n.d.). The success of negotiations also depends on negotiating parties or countries coming to a consensus on the goal of negotiation and how it will be achieved (Meerts, 2015). Negotiation outcomes may be influenced by factors such as the relationship history between negotiating countries, their willingness to make concessions or compromises, and their general attitude or disposition to make a deal (Rodriguez-Garcia, Macinko, Solorzano, & Schlesser, 2001).

The success or failure of negotiations is also primarily driven by political will and the political power to make a deal (Vuković, 2020). Aside from deals brokered at the negotiating table, negotiating parties may still need to confer with political leaders and members of government to convince them to accept the negotiated outcomes (Faizullaev, 2014). Public perception or the acceptance of the negotiating terms can affect whether a deal is acceptable (Rhee, Crabtree, & Horiuchi, 2023). Negotiations may fail if parties believe they can independently achieve their objectives (e.g., through the use of military force) or if one of the sides is unwilling to make any concessions deemed acceptable to the other (Vuković, 2020).

Health as a Bridge for Peace

Health and peace are intricately linked, and it is impossible to have one without the other (Levy 2002). Persistent political and socioeconomic inequalities are often at the heart of conflicts worldwide, and public health issues such as infectious disease outbreaks can be a cause and consequence of war or exacerbate ongoing conflict (Schmidt, 2023). In 2020, the WHO launched the Global Health for Peace Initiative (GHPI) to contribute to the UN SDG Humanitarian-Development-Peace Nexus (WHO.int., 2020). This initiative was designed to "strengthen the role of WHO and the health sector as contributors to improving the prospects for peace – for example, by strengthening social cohesion, dialogue, or resilience to violence" (WHO.int., 2020). Its objectives aim to improve the health and well-being of people living in fragile contexts or areas of past or ongoing conflict (WHO.int., 2020).

Similarly, the theme of the 75th World Health Assembly called for "Health for Peace and Peace for Health" for a healthy and peaceful planet (WHO.int, 2022). The

WHA Member States acknowledged the widening inequalities, global conflict, climate crisis, and calamitous effects of the COVID-19 pandemic on health (WHO.int, 2022). On October 12, 2023, the WHO Executive Board approved a draft resolution demanding" immediate, sustained and unimpeded" humanitarian relief and a humanitarian corridor to allow for transportation of health personnel, patients, medical equipment, and supplies to and from the Gaza strip, amid the Israel-Palestinian war (WHO.int., 2023). The resolution emphasized health as a universal and overarching priority and the promotion of healthcare and human welfare as bridges for peacebuilding (WHO.int., 2023).

Bilateral and Multilateral Collaboration

Global Health Diplomacy is mainly performed through bilateral and multilateral collaborations. Bilateral engagements involve diplomatic efforts and negotiations between two countries intending to forge partnerships for advancing global health priorities (Tago, 2017). Global Health Diplomacy actors can leverage these interactions to lay the groundwork for multilateral diplomacy. Multilateralism rests on the understanding that countries can work collaboratively to achieve a common objective without renouncing their sovereignty (Tago, 2017). Multilateral diplomatic efforts involve multi-country negotiations and can be achieved through international organizations and forums (OGA, 2023). Some examples of multilateral organizations include the World Health Organization, the United Nations, the European Commission, the Group of Twenty (G20), and the Group of Seven (G7) (European Commission, 2022). These international bodies hold summits or conferences that bring together Global Health Diplomacy Actors from multiple nations to develop international agreements, resolutions, policies, or guidelines addressing global health challenges (European Commission,

2022). A key example of multilateral cooperation is the development of the Pandemic Fund. Amongst other objectives, the Pandemic Fund is designed to incentivize countries to increase and secure resources specifically for pandemic prevention, preparedness, and response efforts.

The History of the International Health Regulations

The principal aim of the International Health Regulations is to "prevent, protect against, control and provide a public health response to the international spread of disease to avoid unnecessary interference and international traffic and trade" (WHO, 2005). The International Health Regulations (IHR) can be traced back to International Sanitary Conferences held between 1851 and 1938 that sought to prevent Cholera and other major infectious diseases at the time from spreading into Europe from Asia (WHO, n.d.).

In 1969, the World Health Assembly first adopted the International Health Regulations to prevent the spread of six infectious diseases. In 1973 and 1981, the IHR were amended to refocus its scope on preventing Cholera, Yellow Fever, and the Plague (WHO, n.d.). The subsequent regulations that emerged from these conferences were principally designed to quarantine infected persons in the locations of the outbreaks to shield European countries from these infections (Gostin & Katz, 2016). The emergence and re-emergence of some infectious diseases and global threats, coupled with growing transnational trade and travel, warranted significant revision of these regulations in 1995. These revisions expanded the IHR's scope to include a broader range of diseases and public health threats, including those of biological, chemical, radiological, or nuclear origin, potentially affecting human health (WHO, n.d.).

The revised regulations were adopted on May 23, 2005, at the 58th World Health

Assembly, entered into force for most parties on June 15, 2007, and required that States

Parties inform the WHO of wide-ranging health events (WHO.int, n.d.). The revised

regulations also demanded that State Parties evaluate their surveillance and response

capacity to health threats as part of their implementation milestones and develop and

implement action plans to ensure these essential capacities were fully operational by 2012

(WHO.int, n.d.). Negotiations are ongoing among the World Health Assembly member

states to amend the IHRs to better align with the demands of future pandemics (Cullinan,

2023).

Integrating Health in All Policies for More Equitable Health Outcomes

Considering the multidimensional pathways through which policy across different

sectors affects health, assessing the impact of policies and programs on health outcomes

is imperative (Green et al., 2021). Population health cuts across economic, trade, and

foreign policy, requiring political will and a whole-of-government approach that

transcends the health sector alone (Rudolph, Caplan, Ben-Moshe, & Dillon, 2013). The

Health in All Policies (HiAP) approach aims at integrating health into all public policies

across all sectors (WHO, 2014). This approach recommends a multi-sectorial

consideration for health in decision-making processes and that policymakers seek out

synergies to mitigate harmful effects on health, promote health equity, and improve

population health (WHO, 2014). The World Health Organization defines health inequities

as "the differences in health status or in the distribution of health resources between

different population groups, arising from the social conditions in which people are born,

grow, live, work and age" (WHO, 2018). These inequities are linked to social and structural health determinants, resulting in disparities in the availability, affordability, and accessibility of healthcare, leading to poor health outcomes (WHO, 2018).

Health in All Policies recognizes that humanity's most significant health challenges, such as health inequities and inequalities, non-communicable diseases, climate change, and the rising cost of healthcare, are complex and linked to the social and structural determinants of health (Rudolph, Caplan, Ben-Moshe, & Dillon, 2013).

Equity can only be achieved in the absence of unjust, avoidable, and remediable differences amongst population groups, allowing them to reach their full potential for health and well-being (WHO, 2018). The global disease burden rests principally in the Sub-Saharan African and South Asia regions that host the majority of previously colonized low-and-middle-income countries (Roser, Ritchie, & Spooner, 2021). Several years post-independence, these countries still deal with the legacy of trauma, crippling economic crisis, political instability, and erasure that culminate in persistent inequities stemming from the colonial era (Czyzewski, 2011).

The long history of structural inequity has directly or indirectly plunged these countries into cyclical poverty, poor health outcomes, lack of health infrastructure, reduced quality of life, and decreased life expectancy (Health.gov., n.d.). For example, in sub-Saharan Africa, about 16,000 children die each day from easily preventable infectious diseases (WHO, 2018). The probability of a child in this region dying before their fifth birthday is 14 times greater than in other parts of the world (WHO, 2018). While health inequities existed before COVID-19, they were exacerbated by the pandemic (Moyer et al., 2022). Data from the World Bank's 2022 Poverty and Shared Prosperity Report reveals that over 75 million more people now face extreme poverty (living on less than $1.5 per day), which increases their vulnerability to disease, hunger, and domestic violence (World Bank Group 2022).

Promoting individual, community, and population health in this context requires equitable economic, social, political, environmental, legal, and technological policies (Maani et al., 2023). Regrettably, considerations for health and equity do not always gain precedence during governments' agenda-setting processes amid other competing priorities (WHO, 2018c). Present-day health is shaped by powerful forces such as globalization, climate change, rapid urbanization, and demographic changes (WEF, 2023; EPA, 2021).

Multisectoral collaboration may involve conflicts of interest that warrant innovative solutions and structures that foster dialogue across government agencies, break down siloes, and mitigate unintended harmful health impacts (WHO, 2018c). Although better living conditions may have resulted in the disappearance of some diseases from certain parts of the world, many poverty-related diseases remain prevalent in developing countries (Ramirez-Rubio et al., 2019).

Leveraging One Health to Increase Health Security

The One Health Approach recognizes the close connections between human and animal health and their shared environment (CDC.gov, 2023). The continuous growth and expansion of human populations into new geographic areas have brought them closer to domestic and wild animals, including pets and livestock (Wolf, 2015). For centuries, animals have played an integral role in human societies through nourishment, livelihood, clothing, education, travel, sport, and companionship. Being in close contact with animals increases the probability of disease transmission between humans and animals

(Adisasmito et al., 2022). In addition, increases in climatic variations and land use, including intensive agricultural practices and deforestation, have disrupted natural habitats and environmental conditions that favor the transmission of zoonotic infections to humans (One Health Commission, 2022). Globalization has also increased the movement of people and animals and transnational trade, favoring opportunities for the rapid spread of diseases across borders and around the world (Faustino et al., 2022). A strategic One Health approach is imperative for addressing the knowledge, skills, and capacity gaps by ensuring multisectoral collaboration among scientists, decision-makers, and all stakeholders (Jeggo, Arabena, & Mackenzie, 2019). Thus, for optimal pandemic preparedness planning, disease surveillance, and early warning systems should include operational provisions for identifying and rapidly containing and controlling zoonotic risks before they are introduced to humans (Lefrançois et al., 2023).

Figure 2
One Health Model

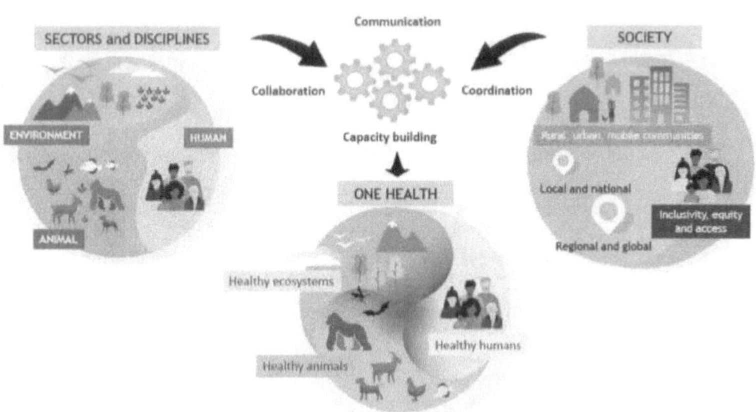

(Adisasmito et al., 2022).

Global Health Diplomacy in Response to the COVID-19 Pandemic

Despite several decades of warnings of global pandemic threats and contingency planning, the United States and the rest of the world were largely unprepared for the COVID-19 pandemic (Frutos, Gavotte, Serra-Cobo, Chen, & Devaux, 2021). An Independent Taskforce Report by the Council of Foreign Relations states: "The COVID-19 pandemic laid bare these failures in global and US domestic preparedness and implementation, exposing important lessons that had not been learned, critical initiatives left unfunded, and solemn obligations that had not been met" (Bollyky & Patrick, 2020). One key lesson from the pandemic is the importance of preparedness anchored in robust surveillance, early warning, and early detection systems for rapid and inclusive deployments and response (Williams, Jones, Welch, & True, 2023).

At the height of the pandemic, the US Secretary of State and the Secretary of HHS jointly proposed four crucial global health security priorities (Blinken & Becerra, 2021). These actions required diplomatic engagements from the US government and collaboration with other international leaders to make the world safer from future pandemics and included the following:

1. Modernizing global institutions like the World Health Organization, UN agencies, and regional and international multilateral financial institutions that have provided funding or funding oversight of emergency preparedness and response. This endeavor warranted reassessing existing roles, resources, and capabilities to respond to global health threats rapidly and effectively.

2. Strengthening pre-existing international regulations, agreements, and norms in line with the changes and demands of the 21st century. These included the effect

of climate change on infectious disease, protection for intellectual property, the development and use of modern technology, and the importance of real-time data and information-sharing.

3. Mobilizing dedicated and sustained financing to support preparedness, prevention, early detection, and response to biological threats. In addition to strengthening countries' health and laboratory systems and funding research and development of new treatments in anticipation of future pandemic responses.

4. Strengthening global leadership and governance anchored in transparency and accountability for developing policies that address systemic equities and inequalities, particularly for populations at greater health risk. Tailored policies and approaches must be designed and adapted for countries of all income levels instead of the wealthiest people being prioritized by default (Blinken & Becerra, 2021).

Initial Assessments of the COVID-19 Aftermath

As of March 2024, the WHO has recorded almost 774 million confirmed COVID-19 cases, with the United States currently registering the highest mortality rate from the virus, with over 1.2 million deaths (WHO.int, 2024). While some COVID-19 databases currently report over 7 million COVID deaths (Worldometer, 2024), the WHO estimates the excess mortality rate (the number of COVID-19 deaths directly or indirectly linked to COVID-19) is around 20 million (WHO.int, 2022). Stoto et al., 2022 analyzed the US excess mortality rates between January 3, 2020, and September 26, 2021, based on 895,693 reported COVID-19 deaths. Their results revealed an excess of 26% more deaths than was initially announced (Stoto, Schlageter, & Kraemer, 2022). Indirect COVID-19-

related deaths result from people's inability to access treatment and prevention during the pandemic due to an overburdened health system and society (WHO.int, 2022).

The disruption and destabilization of lives and livelihoods from COVID-19 and the burden of morbidity and mortality have been so significant that it will take several years for the actual toll of the pandemic to be fully understood and evaluated (World Bank Group, 2023). The emerging disequilibrium between existing and future models and systems and how they adapt and respond to the pandemic aftermath has come under scrutiny in light of these emerging transnational challenges. Over the past three years, the discrepancies between the needs, demands, and the ability of organizations and systems to meet them have been apparent. These challenges have led to significant restructuring as nations and systems grapple with the COVID-19 aftermath, and the field of Global Health Diplomacy is no exception (Shrestha et al., 2020).

Defying the Cycle of Panic and Neglect

Over the years, global health crises have suffered from a cycle of "panic and neglect." This phase is typically characterized by a marked surge in funding and resources in the face of a serious health threat, followed by a chronic funding deficiency toward preparedness for future outbreaks once the news headline moves on (World Bank Group, 2017).

The last four years have reaffirmed how intricately linked health is to every facet of humanity's existence, making COVID-19 not just a health crisis but a universal economic and security crisis as well (World Bank Group, 2023). Within a short period, the virus shut down global economies, trade, and international travel. A 2020 report on the global security impact of COVID-19 reiterated that the virus has "had a profound impact on peace and security across the globe, compounding geopolitical and security challenges, undermining social cohesion and fueling unrest, conflict, violent extremism, populism and disinformation" (UN.org, 2020). In the words of UN Secretary-General Antonio Guterres, "the world faces security challenges that no single country or organization can address alone" (UN.org, 2020).

As devastating as COVID-19 has been, scientific evidence and disease modeling point toward another imminent pandemic or Disease X (Tahir et al., 2021); it is no longer about if another health threat emerges but when (Baker et al., 2021). For instance, a novel influenza virus outbreak could potentially be much worse than COVID-19, resulting in a much higher death toll and even more significant damage to global economies and societies (Barber, 2023).

On May 5, 2023, the Director-General (DG) of the World Health Organization declared "with great hope that COVID-19 was no longer a global health emergency" (UN.org, 2023). This statement was released almost three and a half years after the pandemic had been declared a Public Health Emergency of International Concern (PHEIC) (Torner, 2023). The announcement was made amidst calls for ongoing vigilance, considering the resurgence of cases, recent deaths, and the risk of the emergence of new viral strains (Wise, 2023). With a death toll of approximately 20 million, the DG cautioned, "The worst thing any country could do now is to use this news as a reason to let down its guard, to dismantle the systems it has built, or to send the message to its people that COVID-19 is nothing to worry about." (Wise, 2023). Similarly, on May 11, 2023, the US HHS Secretary, Xavier Becerra, declared the end of the Public Health Emergency phase of the pandemic in the US, citing a 95% decline in COVID-19 deaths and a 91% decrease in hospitalization rates (HHS.gov, 2023).

As was seen in past epidemics like Ebola, a decline in morbidity and mortality rates ushers in the cycle of panic and neglect fueled by diminished political focus and relaxing public health measures, leading to broad misperceptions that the pandemic is over (Jenkins, 2023). The total number of COVID-19 infections continues to rise steadily across the world. In the 28 days between July 24 and August 20, 2023, WHO recorded about 1.5 million new COVID-19 cases and over 200 deaths across its six regions (WHO.int, 2023). In the US, the CDC warned of a late summer wave of COVID-19 infections, reporting 324 deaths and a 21.6% increase in hospital admissions between August 19 and August 24, 2023 (CDC.gov, 2023). With the emergence of the highly mutated variant BA.2.86 in the US and worldwide, the COVID-19 pandemic is far from over (Galvão, 2023; Fauci, 2022). As of March 11, 2024, there were 703 million confirmed COVID-19 infections and over 22 million active COVID-19 cases worldwide, 997,363 of which were recorded in the United States (Worldometer, 2024). As of March 2, 2024, the CDC reported 15,141 weekly new COVID-19 hospital admissions in the US (CDC.gov. 2024).

The Pandemic Fund

The Pandemic Fund is a financing initiative launched by the World Bank in November 2022 to provide sustained multilateral funding for epidemic and pandemic prevention, preparedness, and response (PPPR) (The World Bank, 2023). A G20 High-Level Independent Panel proposed this initiative in response to multiple calls for increased global collaboration and the need for additional international funding to bolster

pandemic preparedness and response capabilities worldwide (WHO, 2022). The
Pandemic Fund aims to purposefully finance critical PPR investments at the national and
regional levels, focusing on low- and middle-income nations. The World Bank and the
World Health Organization estimate an annual pandemic preparedness funding gap of
about 10 billion US Dollars (USAID.gov, 2023).

**The Relevance of Global Health Diplomacy: Research Contribution and
Implications for Practice in a Post-COVID Era**

COVID-19 was a firm reminder of the importance of a multisectoral global health
agenda (Blinken, 2023). As mentioned earlier, health cuts across each country's political,
socio-cultural, and economic landscape. Thus, Global Health Diplomacy is central to
promoting health and addressing diverse global health threats, including infectious and
non-communicable diseases, climate change, health inequities, food security, and the
environment.

This study is timely; it aligns with the critical mission of the new Bureau of
Global Health Security and Diplomacy of elevating global health security as a core US
foreign policy priority (Blinken, 2023). The Bureau will achieve its mission by engaging
in and maintaining purposeful, goal-oriented diplomatic relations with its international
and domestic counterparts to tackle shared global health security challenges (State.gov,
2023).

Launching a New Bureau of Global Health Security and Diplomacy (GHSD)

On December 13, 2022, the US Secretary of State, Antony Blinken, announced
the establishment of a Global Health Security and Diplomacy Bureau as a critical

component of US foreign policy and national security (State.gov, 2022). The new Bureau, which launched on August 1, 2023, is tasked with fostering collaboration between diplomats and health security experts to strengthen global health security to efficiently and effectively prevent, detect, and address current and future health security challenges, including HIV/AIDS (State.gov, 2023).

The Bureau of GHSD embodies the Biden-Harris Administration's dedication to "prioritize global health security as a critical component of national biodefense" (White House.gov, 2023), as well as the Department of State's commitment to advancing human health by protecting US citizens and the rest of the world from health threats (State.gov, 2023).

On January 24, 2024, the Department of State launched a new Lateral Entry Pilot Program (LEPP) designed to recruit 35 mid-career professionals with critical skills and experience from the public and private sectors, academia, and the civil service into the Foreign Service (State.gov, 2024). This initiative demonstrates the Department of State's commitment to strengthening US Foreign Policy priority areas, including "global health security and diplomacy, cyberspace, and emerging technologies; climate, environment, and energy; strategic competition with the People's Republic of China (PRC); economic statecraft; multilateral diplomacy; and consular management" (State.gov., 2024). These efforts are part of the US government and other foreign ministries' efforts to build out their workforce.

The study findings will inform the further development of Georgetown University's Health Diplomacy Training Initiative to build the capacity of formal and informal GHD actors, making them more fit for the practice of Global Health Diplomacy in a post-COVID era.

The Role of Global Health Diplomacy Actors during the COVID-19 Pandemic

Global Health Diplomacy actors were critical in the pandemic response, as they have been in the past (WHO.int, n.d.). For example, international agreements focusing on the global governance of disease and climate, such as the International Health Regulations, the Paris Climate Agreement, and the Framework Convention on Tobacco Control, are classic examples of Global Health Diplomacy outcomes (Meerts, 2015). Responding to COVID-19 required complex, multilevel, multisectoral interactions between state actors, intergovernmental and non-governmental organizations, civil society organizations, public-private partnerships, and sometimes non-state actors (Kickbusch & Liu, 2022).

Table 2

Global Health Diplomacy actors during the COVID-19 pandemic

GHD Domain	Examples	Role
Diplomatic Engagements	Ambassadors, Health Attaches, Consulate Officers, Foreign Affairs Ministers	Facilitated dialogue, negotiations, collaboration, and cooperation between countries to strengthen global health security and advance global health priorities.
International Organizations	The World Health Organization, United Nations, World Bank, Organization for Economic Cooperation and Development, European Commission, etc.	Championed global solidarity, provided technical expertise, public health guidance, and resource coordination to address pandemic-related challenges and allow equitable access for all.
Governance	Leadership at the sub-national, national, and international levels, e.g., Heads of Government Agencies, Ministers of Health, etc.	Set global health priorities, mobilized financial, human, and material resources, and fostered collaboration and coordination of pandemic response efforts.

Multilateral Platforms	Global health summits and conferences, e.g., Group of Seven (G7), Group of Twenty (G20), UN Climate Change Conference, UN General Assembly	Brought together diverse multilevel, multisectoral stakeholders for dialogue, knowledge-sharing, resource mobilization, and the development of joint strategies to respond to the pandemic and address its effects on sustainable development goals.
Civil Society Engagement	Civil Society Organizations, Non-Governmental Organizations (NGOs), International NGOs, e.g., COVAX (CEPI, WHO, and GAVI in partnership with UNICEF to accelerate the development and manufacture of COVID-19 vaccines), Advocacy Groups, Community-based Organizations	Provided grassroots perspectives, mobilized public support and adherence to public health regulations, championed COVID-19 testing and vaccination, and held governments accountable to commitments made to their citizens.
Research and Academia	Research and Academic institutions and networks, e.g., The Center for Global Health Science and Security.	Generated, synthesized, and evaluated evidence. Critically analyzed policies and made recommendations that informed diplomatic negotiations, decision-making, and innovations during the pandemic.
Public-Private Partnerships	Operation Warp Speed (US Government's initiative to speed up COVID-19 vaccine production), the World Economic Forum, Chambers of Commerce.	Fostered collaboration between the public and private sector. The private sector brought expertise, resources, and innovative approaches to addressing the pandemic as per governments' regulatory frameworks and policy guidelines to minimize economic disruptions to global businesses and supply chains.
Technology and Innovation	District Health Information Software (DHIS2), COVID-19 data hosting platforms, Telehealth platforms, Contract-tracing and COVID-19 exposure applications, Artificial Intelligence, Smart Thermometers, etc.	Improved multi-country data collection, surveillance, and timely communication. Enhanced collaboration and knowledge-sharing among multiple stakeholders.

The United States Involvement in Global Health

The United States has demonstrated its vested interest in global health for over a century by actively engaging in international health activities (KFF, 2022). The US commitment to improving the health outcomes of low- and middle-income populations has solidified its status as the most significant donor and implementer of health programs globally. In fiscal year (FY) 2022, the US awarded approximately $12.1 billion to fund global health interventions through bilateral and multilateral partnerships (KFF, 2022) and 13 billion the following year (KFF, 2023). These amounts were more than twice the total spent in FY 2006, excluding supplemental funding for emergency response to Zika, Ebola, and COVID-19 (KFF, 2022).

Figure 3
US Global Health Funding (in millions), By Sector, F.Y. 2023

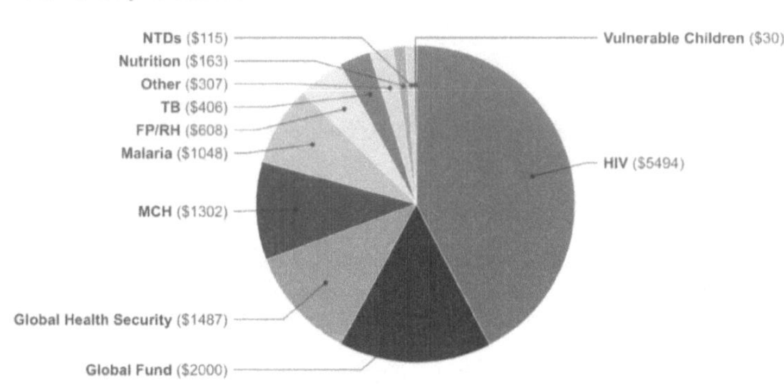

Source:

Concurrently, the US also contributes to foreign policy priorities, national security concerns, and broader development goals. These efforts and more are realized through a

Whole-of-Government approach that leverages multiple US Government agencies and departments, congressional committees, and funding committees.

The United States' multifaceted role in global health includes providing financial, health-related, and development assistance, program operations, health service delivery, emergency and disaster responses, strategic partnering with bilateral, multilateral, and private sector actors, and global health diplomacy (KFF, 2022). The US global health efforts are implemented mainly through agencies and departments within the Executive branch through the Department of State (DOS), the Department of Health and Human Services (HHS), the United States Agency for International Development (USAID), and the Centers for Disease Control and Prevention (CDC) (KFF, 2022).

The Legislative branch or Congress also plays a critical role in the US global health efforts by outlining the US global health priorities and allocating funding to respective US agencies and departments to implement, oversee, and evaluate the impact of these efforts (KFF, 2022).

The United States Whole-of-Government Response to COVID-19

A Whole-of-Government approach is defined as "the movement from isolated silos in public administration to formal and informal networks, driven by various societal forces such as the growing complexity of problems that call for collaborative responses" (UN.org, 2012). This approach seeks to transform how the government serves its people by making public services more effective and accessible, using an equitable, participatory, human-centered design in intervention planning, implementation, and evaluation (Danaa, 2023). These actions can support government efforts to protect the most vulnerable to disease, such as children and the elderly, promote communal and national stability, and ultimately save lives (OECD, 2023).

The US whole-of-government approach to COVID-19 leveraged several federal departments' and government agencies' expertise, capabilities, and resources for a unified and integrated pandemic response (State.gov, 2023). The White House worked through its COVID Task Force to lead and coordinate response efforts, enhance bilateral and multilateral collaboration to strengthen health systems, and improve surveillance, data, and resource sharing (NARA, 2020). The White House also played a central role in setting domestic policies, guidelines, and public health measures to mitigate the virus's rapid spread. Many of these efforts were executed through the Department of Health and Human Services (HHS), the Centers for Disease Control and Prevention (CDC), the National Institutes of Health (NIH), the Federal Emergency Management Agency (FEMA), and the Food and Drug Administration (FDA) in coordination with state and local governments (FEMA, 2020; HHS.gov, n.d.). This approach sought to rapidly control the spread of the virus, ensure the timely and equitable distribution of essential resources, and mitigate its public health impact (DOD, 2020).

The Intelligence Community supported the CDC's and HHS's disease surveillance efforts, monitored and analyzed global data to understand the virus's origin, track its spread in real-time, and assess potential threats to inform the White House's decision-making (Thomas, n.d.). The Intelligence Community is also tasked with gathering and evaluating foreign intelligence relating to foreign governments' or foreign organizations' intentions, capabilities, or activities (DeVine, 2020). The Department of Defense rapidly deployed military personnel to bolster contact tracing, testing, and vaccination efforts and to provide logistical support in setting up emergency field hospitals and mobile laboratories, contributing to surveillance efforts (DOD, 2023). The US Department of Agriculture worked to strengthen cross-disciplinary One Health capacities by providing information, research, and programs on food safety, plant, and animal health for disease prevention (USDA.gov., n.d.). Federal and non-federal essential and frontline workers provided round-the-clock care to the sick, many of whom required intensive care, and ensured ongoing operations of essential services (Blau, Koebe, & Meyerhofer, 2020).

One of the most significant achievements of this whole-of-government approach was securing funding to accelerate research, development, and procurement of vaccines and therapeutics to guarantee vaccine access to everyone within the US (NARA, 2020).

The United States Whole-of-Government Approach to Addressing Global Health Challenges

The United States also leverages the whole-of-government approach to mobilize pooled resources to address transnational global health issues (OECD, 2023).

The Global Health Security Agenda

The Global Health Security Agenda (GHSA) is an example of a whole-of-government effort to address worldwide health security threats. In collaboration with over 70 other countries, the United States seeks to leverage multisectoral partnerships between international organizations and key interested parties from civil society and non-governmental organizations to strengthen global health security (GHSA, 2023). First instituted in 2014, the GHSA seeks to increase countries' capacity in infectious disease prevention, detection, and response to achieve the IHR core capacities (WHO, n.d.).

The rapid spread of infectious diseases over the years, including Ebola, Zika, Avian Influenza, COVID-19, antimicrobial resistance, and emerging bacteria and viruses, highlights the urgency for coordination, cooperation, policy development, and decision-making. In support of its joint strategic priorities, the US CDC has directly engaged with partner country governments in health system strengthening and lowering the risk of infectious disease outbreaks (CDC.gov, 2022).

The GHSA 2024's target objective seeks to ensure that over 100 countries increasingly take ownership of global health security efforts to make the world safer (CDC, 2022). Additionally, these countries are required to complete a Joint External Evaluation (JEE) to attain a level of "demonstrated capacity" in a minimum of 5 technical areas. Several discussions around the COVID-19 response have centered around the concept of resilient health systems, broadly describing the preparedness, management, recovery, and learning abilities of health systems during crises such as these (Burau et al., 2022). The JEE helps countries prioritize opportunities that strengthen preparedness and response by identifying the most critical gaps in both human and animal health systems (WHO, 2022). Table 3 below provides key examples of prior and ongoing whole-of-government global health initiatives by the United States Government.

Table 3

Examples of US Whole-of-Government Approach in Global Health

Timeline	Intervention Area	Global Health Initiative	Results Summary
2005 – Present day	Malaria	The President's Malaria Initiative	Over 7.6 million lives were saved, and 1.5 billion malaria infections were prevented in sub-Saharan Africa and Southeast Asia.

2021	Tuberculosis	Global Tuberculosis Control Efforts [USAID & CDC Active TB Program]	About 33,000 health workers were trained, over 3.8 million tuberculosis cases were diagnosed, and 82,000 started treatment.
2003 – Present day	HIV/AIDS	The President's Emergency Plan for AIDS Relief (PEPFAR)	Over 21 million lives were saved, millions of HIV infections were prevented and supported 20 countries in achieving HIV epidemic control.
2021	Global Health Security	Operational capacity strengthening and provision of technical assistance	Improved health security capacity in 50 countries through strategic partnership and support.
2021 – 2023	COVID-19	USA Procurement and delivery of COVID-19 vaccines.	Supported COVID-19 prevention and relief efforts in over 100 countries by increasing COVID-19 vaccine equity and accessibility

Adapted from OECD's Development Cooperation Tools, Insights, Practices (TIPs). Available at:

The Role of an American Global Health Diplomat

At the helm of the new Bureau of Global Health Security and Diplomacy is Ambassador-at-Large Dr. John N. Nkengasong, who serves as US Global AIDS Coordinator and Special Representative for Health Diplomacy. As Senior Bureau Official and Global Health Ambassador, Dr. Nkengasong's principal responsibilities are leading US diplomatic engagement, leveraging and supporting the coordination of US foreign assistance, and promoting multilevel international cooperation to prevent domestic and global health threats (State.gov, 2023). The GHSD Bureau's leadership team supports diplomatic coordination and collaboration within the Department of State, across other

US government agencies, and among US international partners (State.gov, 2023). This group constitutes the Core Global Health Diplomacy actors.

Also, within the category of Core GHD actors are Health Attachés, a specialized cadre of Global Health Diplomats that occupy a pivotal role at the intersection between global health and diplomacy (OGA, 2022). The US Health Attachés interface with foreign Ministries of Health, Science and Technology, support US Embassy personnel, and several divisions within the Department of Health and Human Services (OGA, 2022). Health Attachés facilitate a variety of health-related activities within their host countries, such as pandemic preparedness and response efforts, infectious, emerging, and non-communicable diseases, global health security, and environmental health (OGA, 2022).

The list below highlights some responsibilities Global Health Diplomacy actors may be called upon to perform in a post-COVID era. This list is informed by the role and responsibilities of Health Attachés during the COVID-19 pandemic (OGA, 2022), in addition to those advanced by Brown et al., 2014 and may include:

1. Advocating for global health policies and initiatives that advance health security, promote equitable health access, improve maternal and child health outcomes, and address infectious diseases.
2. Leading diplomatic negotiation and mediation to further US global health interests through international engagement and collaboration.
3. Developing and fostering strategic bilateral and multilateral partnerships and agreements for coordination and resource mobilization to address global health challenges and threats.

4. Representing the United States at international health fora, meetings, and health conferences to articulate the US' priorities and position on various health issues and providing expertise

5. Gathering, synthesizing, analyzing, and disseminating information on global health trends and emerging threats, sharing insights, evidence-based practices, and recommendations of best practices to inform US policy design and decision-making.

6. Coordinating international health emergency efforts, mobilizing resources in response to global health crises, and providing technical assistance to affected countries.

7. Fostering collaboration to build and strengthen partner countries' health, laboratory, and supply chain systems to enhance their ability to respond to health emergencies and disease outbreaks.

Thus, this researcher defines the overarching role of a US Global Health Diplomat in a post-COVID era is to represent the United States in global health-related matters to promote and protect the health, health equity, and well-being of US citizens and the rest of the world. By collaborating with foreign governments, international organizations, and multisectoral stakeholders, US Global Health Diplomats work to advance the US' global health agenda for better health outcomes worldwide.

The Role of Global Health Diplomacy in Foreign Assistance

Beyond health-related matters, Global Health Diplomacy can also serve as the foundation for diplomatic relations across different sectors. For example, the Office of Foreign Assistance oversees and coordinates US foreign aid in the form of money, physical goods, and services lent or gifted to other countries (Office of Foreign

Assistance, 2021). Foreign aid typically falls into three main categories: economic

and development assistance, humanitarian assistance, and security assistance (Office

of Foreign Assistance, 2021). The US has donated nearly 4 trillion dollars since the

Second World War, with almost 50% distributed through USAID (CFR, 2023). Table

4 provides annual funds distributed by the United States to its managing agencies in

2022. Figure 4 details which countries received the most American foreign assistance

that year.

Table 4

2022 US Foreign Assistance Disbursement Per Managing Agency

Managing Agency	Funds Disbursed in 2022
US Agency for International Development	$38.7188 billion
Department of State	$21.3531 billion
Department of the Treasury:	$2.59726 billion
Department of Health and Human Services	$2.16256 billion
Department of Defense	$1.95385 billion
Millennium Challenge Corporation	$692.234 million
Peace Corps	$387.712 million
Department of Agriculture	$307.117 million
Department of Energy	$192.895 million
Department of the Interior	$168.515 million

Adapted from Foreignassistance.gov dashboard. Available at:
https://www.foreignassistance.gov/

Figure 4

Top recipient countries of US foreign aid in 2022

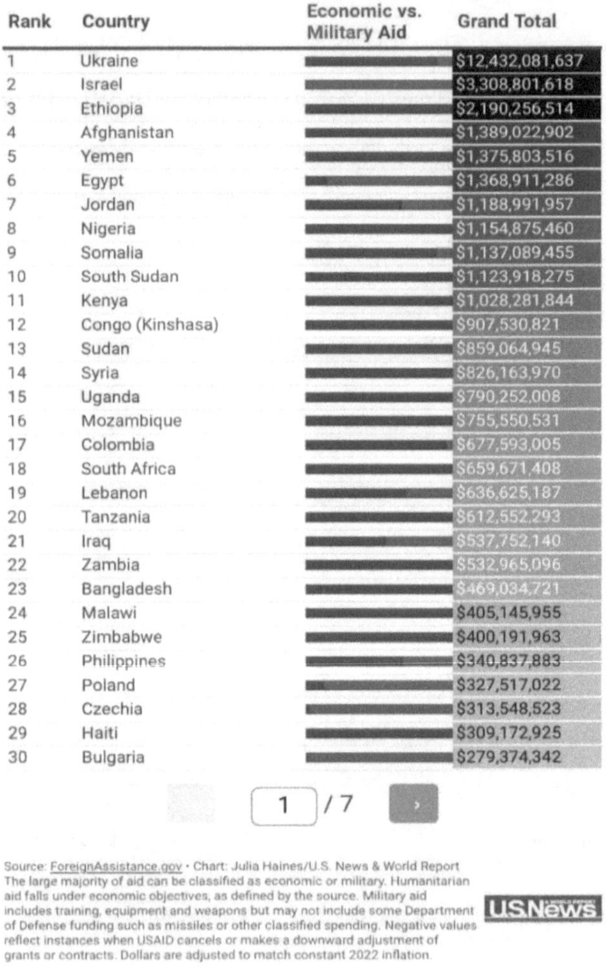

Rank	Country	Economic vs. Military Aid	Grand Total
1	Ukraine		$12,432,081,637
2	Israel		$3,308,801,618
3	Ethiopia		$2,190,256,514
4	Afghanistan		$1,389,022,902
5	Yemen		$1,375,803,516
6	Egypt		$1,368,911,286
7	Jordan		$1,188,991,957
8	Nigeria		$1,154,875,460
9	Somalia		$1,137,089,455
10	South Sudan		$1,123,918,275
11	Kenya		$1,028,281,844
12	Congo (Kinshasa)		$907,530,821
13	Sudan		$859,064,945
14	Syria		$826,163,970
15	Uganda		$790,252,008
16	Mozambique		$755,550,531
17	Colombia		$677,593,005
18	South Africa		$659,671,408
19	Lebanon		$636,625,187
20	Tanzania		$612,552,293
21	Iraq		$537,752,140
22	Zambia		$532,965,096
23	Bangladesh		$469,034,721
24	Malawi		$405,145,955
25	Zimbabwe		$400,191,963
26	Philippines		$340,837,883
27	Poland		$327,517,022
28	Czechia		$313,548,523
29	Haiti		$309,172,925
30	Bulgaria		$279,374,342

1 / 7 >

Source: US News & World Report. Available at: https://www.usnews.com/news/best-countries/articles/countries-that-receive-the-most-foreign-aid-from-the-u-s

As the world's largest humanitarian aid donor, the United States has maintained a steady role in the health, aid, and development sectors. For over sixty years, the US Agency for International Development (USAID) has provided critical multisectoral disaster assistance through strategic partnerships and investments that save lives, promote democracy, and alleviate poverty (USAID, 2023). This aid has provided much-needed nutrition, water and sanitation, food, emergency shelter, cash, livelihood support, child protection, and prevention of gender-based violence. This assistance has also supported the recovery of vulnerable populations after natural and man-made disasters beyond humanitarian aid (USAID, 2022).

The diplomatic influence of the US has been evident in its active and ongoing response to conflict, international disasters, and the protection of refugees and vulnerable populations (USAID.gov, 2022). Through active diplomatic negotiations, collaboration, and advocacy, the US Department of State and USAID strive to ensure the respect of humanitarian principles within US foreign policy and protect at-risk populations, including victims of conflict, internal displacement, and forced migration (USAID.gov, 2022).

Achieving and sustaining durable solutions requires a holistic approach across their diplomatic, development, and relief efforts and effective linkages between health, humanitarian, development, and security programs.

Emerging US Global Health Security and Diplomacy Priorities for 2024

Global health security remains a top national security priority for the United States as it strives to stop infectious disease threats at its source to help forestall the next global pandemic (White House.gov, 2023). The *Global Health Security Partnerships Annual Progress Report* released by the White House on December 30, 2023, accentuated the results of the US's ongoing investments in global health security efforts (White House.gov, 2023). The United States. is committed to providing dedicated resources through political, technical, and financial support to develop, enhance, and maintain effective global health security capacities by strengthening health systems in 50 countries (White House.gov, 2023). These investments will support outbreak prevention, detection, response, and recovery efforts to global health threats, eventually saving trillions of dollars and preventing the loss of millions of lives (White House.gov, 2023).

The year 2024 marks an inflection point in the global health security and diplomacy landscape for the United States and the rest of the world. Below are a few of the Biden Administration's top priorities for which the US seeks to galvanize multilateral engagement and collaboration to foster global security and solidarity (White House.gov, 2023).

- Strengthening and sustaining the Global Health Security Agenda beyond 2024 by ensuring continuous technical support, multilateral and multisectoral collaborations, and measuring stakeholder accountability against set targets.
- Continuous support of financial commitment and contributions to the World Bank's Pandemic Fund for global pandemic preparedness efforts, especially in countries and regions with the direst needs, most significant capacity, and operational gaps.

- Accelerate progress towards the G7 Pact for Pandemic Readiness milestones to support financing pandemic preparedness endeavors and response for 100 countries in collaboration with Italy's G7 and Brazil's G20 presidencies.

- Strengthening the framework of global health security through ongoing negotiations of the International Health Regulations amendment and developing a Pandemic Agreement ahead of the next World Health Assembly in May 2024 (White House.gov, 2023).

To deliver on these priorities, members of the GHSD Bureau plan to partner with multisectoral leadership from all facets of the community, leverage financial investments for health security, outbreak prevention, and response, and elevate health security within all countries' foreign policy agendas (Carter & Bollyky, 2024).

Training Recommendations for GHD Professionalization or Strengthening

The table below presents recommendations from 16 peer-reviewed journal articles published between 2019 and 2024 that specifically addressed either knowledge, skills, or competencies of Global Health Diplomacy in line with current and future global health security threats and priorities. The training recommendations span several domains to strengthen the public health workforce and GHD actors' capacity in pandemic preparedness, prevention, and response. Some studies highlighted the need for a refresher and more frequent training, as well as updating training curricula for medical and public health schools in alignment with inadequacies highlighted by the recent pandemic. The table below presents the knowledge, skills, and competencies of Global Health Diplomats based on key literature.

Table 5

Knowledge, Skills, and Competencies of Global Health Diplomats According to the Literature

Training Recommendations for GHD Professionalization or Strengthening GHD Actors' Capacity	Author/Reference
Strengthen health system resilience by training the health workforce in planning, organization, rapid adaption, and transformation amid the rising and changing demands of health services.	(Burau et al., 2022) (Biddle, Wahedi, & Bozorgmehr, 2020)
Develop and master advanced digital communication skills to generate engaging social media content, edit, and ethically promote information, and explore more efficient healthcare models to reach multiple audiences effectively.	(Gasparyan et al., 2022)
Strengthen multisectoral diplomacy, negotiation, advocacy, coalition-building, strategic partnership development, and conflict management skills to navigate political relations, support priority-setting, and address multi-level challenges and complexities in preventing and controlling non-communicable diseases (NCDs).	(Asadi-Lari et al., 2021)
Conduct virtual trainings in virus containment, delivered in a low-dose, high-frequency format to build capacity-building and circumvent restrictions imposed by geography, physical distancing measures, and stay-at-home orders. Setting up communities of practice for disseminating information and sharing best practices, tele-mentoring, case-based learning, health promotion, literature reviews, and South-to-South and South-to-North knowledge and experience sharing.	(Talisuna et al., 2022)
Strengthen Local Health Departments' Public Health Workforce skills in assessing and managing change, human resource development and management, communication for external audiences, and performance management within justice, equity, diversity, and inclusion efforts.	(Zemmel et al., 2021).
Review the public health competency framework developed by WHO and ASPHER (The Association of Schools of Public Health in the European Region) to support aligning public health and global health core competencies across multiple sectors. Develop new and transformative public health leadership and governing models, and health workforce changes to break up professional and policy silos and expand the critical public health competencies beyond the core public health workforce to all healthcare professions. Maintain deliberate focus on building resilience and preparedness in emergencies and ensure public health considerations are central to workforce development, education, planning, and policymaking.	(Czabanowska & Kuhlmann, 2021). (WHO.int., 2020).
Reimagine post-pandemic global health education to include innovative, decolonial, flexible, inclusive, and bi-directional training approaches by global health instructors to foster equitable access to educational content for post-pandemic needs. Co-create educational resources, sharing	(Weine et al., 2021)

knowledge on the use of distance learning technology and best practices for developing and maintaining multinational mentorship networks.	
Conduct refresher training to develop new skills mix and competencies, including multi-professional collaboration, teamwork, and public health knowledge. Develop sustainable recruitment and staffing mechanisms, reorganize and realign the health workforce to accommodate population demographic shifts, such as aging, rising NCDs, and growing global health threats. Conduct rapid training on the use of new technology, particularly for remote healthcare delivery.	(Zapata, Buchan, & Azzopardi-Muscat, 2021).
Train Hospital Management in crisis leadership skills, competencies, and traits across transformative, contingency, participative, and transactional crisis leadership domains. Develop analytical/multidimensional thinking, problem-solving, and strategic and operational planning skills to support crisis prevention, preparedness, response, and recovery, multistakeholder partnerships through intentional networking, crisis communication, human resource organization, and motivational team building. Cultivate crisis leadership traits, e.g., courage, confidence, self-assurance, emotional intelligence, urgency, and the ability to tolerate ambiguity.	(Abdi, Lega, & Ravagi, 2021)
Strengthen cross-disciplinary education integrating GHD training into medical and health-related professions such as health leadership, health administration, health policy, and global health to equip health professionals with the required knowledge and skills for multistakeholder engagements and trade policy negotiations.	(Chattu, Pooransingh, & Allahverdipour 2021)
Develop professional training for the public health workforce that includes a combination of managerial competencies and soft skills (prompt and evidence-based decision-making, multidisciplinary team building, accountability, emotional intelligence, building trust, and effective communication).	(Valz Gris et al., 2022)
Train and develop essential skills such as cultural humility, flexibility, resourcefulness, interprofessional communication, an understanding of sociocultural and economic contexts, and social determinants of health through collaboration between trainees from high-income and LMIC countries to better understand health inequities and how to address them.	(Pancheshnikov et al., 2023)
Strategically assess public health training competencies, gleaning examples from public health, health policy, organizational studies, health systems, policy research, and sociology and integrating these public health and global health competencies for innovative health workforce training according to lessons learned, weaknesses, and opportunities from the global COVID-19 response.	(Kuhlmann, Dussault, & Correia, 2021)
Redesign and modernize the medical training curriculum to include a 'whole-educational' approach to health amid the intense focus on acute or curative health services. Incorporate health promotion as an academic discipline for building resilience and preparing medical students and health personnel for future crises.	(Vankova, 2022)

Elevate health promotion as a core competency for health educators and health authorities for more effective campaigns for positive behavior change, increased public health literacy, and stronger disease transmission prevention efforts during pandemics.	(Van den Broucke, 2020)

Proposed Training Domains for Building and Strengthening the Capacity of Global Health Diplomacy Actors

Global Health Diplomacy actors need to be trained to develop critical thinking and build a diverse set of skills, knowledge, and competencies to navigate the intricacies and demands of their roles effectively. The scope, content, and duration of training will vary based on the needs and specificity of the role and responsibilities of GHD actors. For example, the training needs of diplomats, foreign service staff, and public health professionals differ from those of civil society representatives or GHD actors in research and academia.

The proposed domains are informed by the US Government's 2024 global health security and diplomacy priorities, previously referenced research publications, and some multidisciplinary Global Health Diplomacy trainings created between 2019 and 2023. These trainings were designed to build and strengthen GHD actors' ability and capacity to respond to the COVID-19 pandemic and other imminent global health challenges and improve GHD practice by building transferable skills to support GHD practice in diverse settings.

The Global Health Security and Diplomacy Training at Georgetown University is designed to "explore the interconnection between foreign affairs, national security and global health issues such as pandemic preparedness and response and examine the role of diplomacy and policymaking processes in addressing global health issues" (Center for Global Health Science and Security, 2023).

The Global Health Centre Executive Courses at the Geneva Graduate Institute training for health and diplomatic professionals in Global health Diplomacy and global health governance (Geneva Graduate Institute, 2024).

The Executive Course in Global Health Diplomacy at the Dalla Lana School of Public Health designed "for professionals working in health or health-related sectors, this course will explore the theory and practice of global health diplomacy as it relates to COVID-19 and other current health issues" (Dalla Lana School of Public Health, 2023).

The World Health Organization's Leaderships Skills Training on Global Health Policy and Diplomacy 2021 online training program designed to "help key decision-makers in Member States of the Eastern Mediterranean Region work together effectively to develop global health policy" (WHO.int, 2021).

Global Health Diplomacy training launched in 2020 at the Clingendael Academy was designed for diplomats in response to "changing dynamics and accelerated challenges in Global Health Diplomacy as a result of the COVID-19 Pandemic" (Clingendael, 2021).

Some key training areas, as informed by the literature and initial hypothesis, may include:

1. **Diplomacy, statecraft, and foreign policy** training can facilitate constructive dialogue and relationship building. Diplomacy within the scope of this study encompasses all the things Global Health Diplomacy actors do to advocate for their interests and promote their national agendas to the rest of the world (CFR, 2017).

Diplomacy is considered a 'soft power' tool that can be utilized in different circumstances depending on a specific goal. Soft power is a country's ability to influence a desired outcome through attraction and persuasion rather than employing coercive tactics (Nye, 2017). Depending on the desired result, different forms of diplomacy may include bilateral negotiations, consultative meetings between countries to resolve a shared challenge, global summits of conferences, and back-channel conversations amongst countries with ongoing conflict (CFR, 2017).

The competence of Global Health Diplomacy actors can be bolstered through training in different aspects of diplomacy to better prepare them for the demands of their roles and responsibilities that may not always be intuitive. Much of diplomacy takes place through day-to-day interactions between diplomats, their host country officials, and the broader public for a deeper immersion into the host's culture to build or strengthen diplomatic ties. Training can support this process by helping GHD actors navigate the political and cultural sensitivities in GHD practice. It can also equip them to be better mediators during conflict resolution or cease-fire agreement negotiations, leveraging health as a bridge for peace to allow the delivery of critical humanitarian aid and medical supplies amidst ongoing conflict (de Quadros & Epstein, 2002).

2. **Public health** training can confer a strong knowledge and an understanding of global health challenges, emerging health threats, social and structural determinants of health, and public health principles. Social determinants of health (SDOH) are "the conditions in the environments where people are born, live, learn, work, play, worship, and age that affect a wide range of health, functioning, and quality-of-life outcomes and risks" (Healthy People 2030, n.d.). Structural determinants of health

are "the social, economic, and political mechanisms which generate social class inequalities in society" (WHO.int, 2010). To better appraise these subject matters, GHD actors must recognize the global disease burden and seek to understand how these socio-economic, cultural, and environmental factors may contribute to higher morbidity and mortality rates in specific populations (Ariansen, Gloppen, Rakner, Johansson, & Haaland, 2020). In addition to knowledge of epidemiology to help explain the emergence, prevalence, and trends of disease, GHD actors must understand the root causes of health disparities, the workings of the health system, and how an interplay of these factors can negatively affect population health and worsen existing health inequities (Smith & Hanson, 2011).

3. **Policy analysis and advocacy** training can enable GHD actors to understand the global health policymaking process and agenda-setting (CDC Office of Policy, Performance, and Evaluation, 2022). Global Health Diplomacy actors may be required to evaluate several policy options and make recommendations to country leadership based on specific criteria such as feasibility, efficiency, effectiveness, equity, and acceptability (Kingdon, 1995). Global Health Diplomacy actors may also be called upon to interpret policy, defend, or advocate for their proposed policy options. Aligning policy with the most pressing health needs is critical; therefore, understanding this process will equip them to effectively promote and advance key priorities within the global health arena (Michaud & Kates, 2013). They may also assess the proposed policy options' potential financial and economic implications (Kingdon, 1995), as not every strategy will work in every setting and for every population, not even if communities share demographic similarities. Moreover, this

training can help ensure that the voices and perspectives of those directly affected by the policy have been duly considered and incorporated throughout the decision-making process.

4. **Effective leadership and management** training can ensure proper stakeholder coordination and collaboration within the global health arena, particularly in disease outbreaks and emergencies (Reina Ortiz et al., 2021). By nature, global health crises can be unpredictable. Global Health Diplomacy actors must be versed in standard operation procedures of crisis management and be prepared to lead during an emergency. This responsibility may require convening key interest parties for negotiation, multisectoral collaboration, and resource allocation in response to the situation. While a global health crisis concerns everyone, vulnerable and marginalized communities are disparately affected (Weiner, 2020). Globally, underserved and under-resourced communities were the most affected by the COVID-19 pandemic. Therefore, GHD actors must advocate for prioritizing and equitably distributing resources to those who need them most (Davison et al., 2021). Many of these populations constitute the 'last mile' and reside in hard-to-reach areas with limited access to health care and essential health services.

5. **Cultural competence and cross-cultural communication** training can help smooth the way for diverse multistakeholder engagements with counterparts from different cultural backgrounds. Cultural competence is "a set of congruent behaviors, attitudes, and policies that come together in a system, agency or among professionals and enable that system, agency or those professions to work effectively in cross-cultural situations" (NCCC, n.d.). Negotiating health agreements requires forming alliances to

galvanize collective support toward a desired outcome. To build trusted relationships, GHD must demonstrate attitudes and behaviors that value and respect diversity and cultural differences to foster collaboration and dialogue (Biletska, Lastovskyi, & Semchynskyy, 2023). Cultural competence also helps GHD actors be more aware of their own world views and how these may differ from others and helps confer a more rounded outlook when working inter-culturally (Biletska, Lastovskyi, & Semchynskyy, 2023).

6. **Working knowledge of the legal and ethical contexts** of their assignments or operations. The Universal Declaration of Human Rights, proclaimed in 1948, was adopted by the United Nations and champions a life free and void of want and fear for everyone, irrespective of who or where they are (United Nations, 2015). However, the political, social, economic, cultural, and civic realities within countries can infringe on these human rights and freedoms (Hall-Clifford & Cook-Deegan, 2021). It is not uncommon for Global Health Diplomacy actors to work in locations or contexts rife with human rights violations and ethical dilemmas (Hall-Clifford & Cook-Deegan, 2021). Questions about global health ethics span a broad range of topics. These include but are not limited to appropriate disease control measures, States' obligations in providing health care services, and moral issues surrounding sexuality and reproductive health (WHO.int, n.d.). Legal and ethics training can facilitate GHD actors' understanding and consideration of the International Health Regulations that govern these issues and the existing economic and trade agreements and how they might affect global health negotiations.

7. **Data analysis and research** training can help GHD actors accurately synthesize, analyze, and interpret health data. Reliable health data is central to understanding global health trends and the state of health delivery worldwide (WHO.int, n.d.). The insights gleaned from health statistics and research findings can inform policy development, funding priorities, and evidence-based decision-making. This information is also valuable for assessing countries' progress towards the Sustainable Development Goals. The seventeen Sustainable Development Goals were adopted in 2015 by all member states of the United Nations and provide a shared agenda for achieving global peace and prosperity for humans and the planet, now and in the years to come (United Nations, n.d.).

8. **A mastery of written and spoken foreign languages** is essential for effective communication. Training in foreign languages will enable GHD actors to be more attuned to the cultures and contexts in which they operate (Lazzarini, 2015). It can also make them more effective in carrying out the requirements of their roles, such as negotiations and written and oral presentations. Although GHD actors may employ the services of translators or interpreters while engaging with their counterparts who may not speak the GHD actors' first language, communicating in the local language helps forge deeper diplomatic connections (Council of American Ambassadors, n.d.). According to the Former Director of the Foreign Service Institute, "For every challenge, the key to outreach, understanding and impact is the ability to speak directly to people in their own language and the capability to understand local perspectives" (Whiteside, 2008). Languages are a gateway into other cultures and

facilitate a more accurate understanding of what is being said, what the GHD actor

hears, non-verbal cues, and nuances therein.

Proposed Training Methods for Current and Future Global Health Diplomacy Actors

As the field of Global Health Diplomacy evolves to meet growing global health

challenges, the training of GHD actors must also develop and adapt accordingly. Future

GHD training will most likely include a blend of traditional and innovative approaches to

meet the demands of the post-COVID era. Training curricula will require an amalgam of

interdisciplinary education, ongoing professional development, experiential learning and

in-class simulations, technology-enhanced learning, and microlearning or just-in-time

learning.

The proposed approaches are informed by the Global Health Diplomacy Trainings

previously referenced, as well as from training and education adaptations made during

the COVID-19 pandemic and recommendations for a post-pandemic era. In 2020,

UNESCO's International Commission on Futures of Education published '*Education in a

post-COVID world: Nine ideas for Public Action*' for navigating educational challenges

in the pandemic aftermath. This list highlights the importance of public health education,

cooperation, and solidarity for the common good and the need for integrated curricula

tailored to current themes and issues that affect humanity and our shared environment

(UNESCO, 2020).

In 2021, the World Economic Forum also called for reimaging capacity-building

initiatives to keep up with the changes and demands of educational systems in a post-

pandemic era (Yan & Saguine, 2021). Reimaging education will be contingent upon policymakers and multisectoral stakeholders' ability to "clearly picture the promises and pitfalls of new and existing approaches to counter the challenges, such as learning loss or the digital divide, which have been imposed or exacerbated by the pandemic" (Yan & Saguine, 2021). Some proposed adaptations to GHD education and training in a post-COVID era include:

1. **Interdisciplinary education:** The intersection of health with all other facets of humanity will require a broader multidisciplinary approach to future GHD training. This approach must go beyond building public health and foreign policy expertise to include relevant fields such as economics, trade, law, and sociology. Ideally, the training of GHD actors should consist of collaboration and exchange programs between public health and diplomacy schools.

2. **Experiential learning:** Future GHD training programs must combine didactic and experiential learning that allows participants to develop and hone their skills in the real world. Providing GHD actors or trainees with practical experiences such as internships, mentorships, field placements, and real-world simulations (e.g., mock negotiations) will offer hands-on opportunities for them to apply their knowledge.

3. **Technology-enhanced learning:** Technology-enhanced learning uses technology to strengthen students' learning experiences by leveraging online platforms, interactive tools, collaborative workspaces, and virtual simulations. This form of education gives GHD actors and students learning flexibility and accessibility to training materials, irrespective of location. Not only does this allow for increased

participation of people from diverse cultures and backgrounds, but it also furthers the reach and scalability of GHD training programs.

4. **Collaborative partnerships:** Global Health Diplomacy training programs can foster multistakeholder collaboration, knowledge exchange, and learning opportunities between academic institutions, governments, international organizations, and civil society organizations. These partnerships can help strengthen and broaden existing GHD networks, increase data access, and support resource-sharing.

5. **Continuous professional development:** The rapidly changing global health trends and emerging health security threats require that GHD actors continue to develop professionally to keep abreast with these challenges. Future GHD training programs should ideally offer continuous learning opportunities through conferences, workshops, webinars, and satellite presentations during conferences to support the professional demands of GHD practice. For example, microlearning supports content delivery in small, easily digestible formats with specific learning outcomes (Elm Learning, 2023). These types of training typically range between 3-5 minutes, allowing the learner to complete their training just in time or at their convenience.

Research Gaps

The literature review contributes to understanding the knowledge, skills, and core competencies required by Global Health Diplomacy actors in a post-pandemic era. While a significant amount of literature has been published between 2019 and 2024 on GHD challenges and opportunities from the recent pandemic, the researcher did not find any studies that have explicitly focused on all three domains of required knowledge, skills, and competencies across all three GHD actor categories. The diversity of GHD actors underscores the importance of a tailored approach to identifying and filling training needs in GHD actors' knowledge, skills, and core competencies to ensure they are better equipped for GHD practice in a post-COVID era. Therefore, there is a need for more research to bridge this gap, which this study seeks to address.

Chapter Three: Methods

This chapter presents the study's aims, research questions, data collection, analysis, and interpretation approach. The chapter is divided into three main sections: research methodology and study design, data collection, and data analysis.

I. Research Methodology, Study Population, and Study Design

Study Aims and Research Questions

This study investigated the knowledge, skills, and core competencies required by Core, Multistakeholder, and Informal GHD actors to practice Global Health Diplomacy in a post-COVID era. The study's aims and research questions were as follows:

Aim 1: Determine the required skills and core competencies for Global Health Diplomacy practice for each GHD actor role.

The researcher defines "skills" as specific learned abilities required to successfully practice Global Health Diplomacy. The researcher defines "core competencies" as the essential knowledge, skills, and abilities that GHD actors need to effectively practice Global Health Diplomacy and the proper application of these knowledge, skills and abilities at the right place and time. The researcher defines "Global Health Diplomacy Actors" as individuals, government agencies, institutions, organizations, or entities that cultivate interactions and negotiations between and among each other and within and across governments and states, with the principal objective of improving population health.

Research Question 1: What skills do GHD actors need for effective Global Health Diplomacy practice in a post-COVID era?

Research Question 2: What core competencies do GHD actors need for effective Global Health Diplomacy practice in a post-COVID era?

Aim 2: Identify technical knowledge gaps for each Global Health Diplomacy actor category.

The researcher defines "technical knowledge" as the practical or theoretical understanding of Global Health Diplomacy.

Research Question 3: What technical knowledge gaps exist amongst Global Health Diplomacy actors?

Aim 3: Define Global Health Diplomacy in a post-COVID era.

"Define," as used by the researcher, means to describe or explain the meaning of Global Health Diplomacy based on the GHD actor's understanding of knowledge, skills, and competencies required for practice in a post-COVID era.

Research Question 4: How do Global Health Diplomacy actors define Global Health Diplomacy in a post-COVID era?

Aim 4: Generate a summary of core competency requirements for GHD practice in a post-COVID era based on data from each GHD actor level.

The researcher anticipates that this information will be used to inform the development of targeted training for each category of GHD actors.

Study Population

The study population comprised US-based Core, Multistakeholder, and Informal Global Health Diplomacy actors represented in **Figure 1** (Pyramid of Global Health

Diplomacy). This taxonomy was proposed by Katz et al. following their assessment of

the different approaches to Global Health Diplomacy and how these actors influenced

foreign policymaking and international health in an era of globalization (Katz et al.,

2011).

The Global Health Diplomacy actor categories are described in further detail below:

1. **Core Health Diplomacy:** Represented by the top rung of the pyramid, this

   category includes specialized diplomats and Health Attachés. These are members

   of the formal diplomatic corps with the highest level of credentialing associated

   with GHD practice. Their role specificity accounts for the comparatively few

   numbers of actors in this group. Their principal responsibilities include fostering

   interactions between governments, reporting, negotiating, and developing

   agreements between and among states and governments. Some diplomacy tools

   used by this group include bilateral and multilateral treaties and agreements

   between and among government and state actors (Brown et al., 2014).

2. **Multistakeholder Diplomacy:** Represented by the middle rung of the pyramid,

   this category comprises government employees and representatives of multilateral

   organizations. They are responsible for negotiating and facilitating interactions

   between and among state, non-state, and multilateral actors, some of which may

   not be binding. The credentialing standards for this group are more diverse than

   with the Core actors, resulting in a greater number of actors in this category. Tools

   for diplomacy at this level include establishment and sustainability of partnerships

   amongst government agencies and institutions within countries (Brown et al.,

   2014).

3. **Informal Health Diplomacy:** Represented by the base of the pyramid, this

   category also has significant variance in credentialing and the greatest number of

   health diplomacy actors. It encompasses representatives from the private sector,

   non-governmental organizations, civil society organizations, academia,

   government employees, and the public (Brown et al., 2014). This group is

   responsible for interactions between public health actors and their counterparts in

   the field and plays a critical role in a whole-of-society approach to pandemic

   prevention, preparedness, and response by producing and providing information

   that informs program and policy design and implementation (Dubb, 2020). The

   tools for diplomacy include agreements or memoranda of understanding among

   humanitarian organizations, universities, private-sector companies, private

   funders, and the public (Brown et al., 2014).

Grounded Theory, Descriptive Qualitative Research Design

This study employed a Grounded Theory, descriptive qualitative design, that allowed the researcher to "see" the research problem through the "eyes" of GHD practitioners. Qualitative research examines the nature, quality, and different manifestations of contextualized phenomena and how they are perceived (Busetto, Wick, & Gumbinger, 2020). It involves images, language, and other methods of expressing meaning that is interpreted by the researcher (Remler & Van Ryzin, 2015). Grounded Theory facilitated the exploration and presentation of more targeted solutions grounded in the data that emerged from the interviewees' perspectives (Glaser & Strauss, 2017) on the required knowledge, skills, and core competencies for GHD practice in a post-COVID era, thus increasing study validity.

Grounded Theory typically relies on qualitative data from small purposive samples directed toward a novel topic or research angle that has not yet been clearly defined. While significant information about Global Health Diplomacy has existed over the past two centuries, this research focuses on the post-COVID era, which is less than two years old and presents an inflection point in this field. Although much of the recent literature and publications have focused on the relevance of Global Health Diplomacy from the COVID-era, only a few research articles have narrowed in on one or more domains of GHD knowledge, skills, and core competencies required for actors in a post-pandemic period. As such, although Grounded Theory does not provide a conclusive answer to a problem, it helps inform the exact nature of a problem and can be better supported by descriptive research (Glaser & Strauss, 2017). This type of research can be used to develop solutions to complex issues, allowing for the emergence of new ideas or for developing practical, feasible solutions that may be cost-saving in the long term (Glaser & Strauss, 2017; Swedberg, 2020). For example, equipping GHD actors with the required knowledge, skills, and core competencies to deal with health security threats is a key component of strengthening global pandemic preparedness measures and requires significantly less time and resources than a pandemic response.

Descriptive research "expands knowledge of a project or phenomenon by describing it according to its characteristics or concerning the population to answer the questions of what, when, and how but not the why" (Skidmore, 2022). While descriptive research focuses on present phenomena, including viewpoints, trends, beliefs, or perceptions of the study population, it can also be used for previous events that inform or affect current conditions (Glaser & Strauss, 2017). Thus, this integrated Grounded

Theory, descriptive research design leverages both the exploratory strengths of Grounded Theory and descriptive research methods. Study participants' descriptions and explanations of the knowledge, skills, and core competencies for GHD practice in a post-COVID era provided direct insights into their roles, responsibilities, and expectations for other GHD actors. Their responses also shed light on the diversity and specificity of the roles of GHD actors, which will be utilized in informing training for current and future GHD practitioners.

Rationale for Research Design

This research design adopts a pragmatic approach (Neergaard et al., 2009) to study concepts to guide decision-making in the research process, thus facilitating the selection of the most appropriate methods to answer the research questions (Bishop, 2015). According to Ramanadhan et al., a pragmatic approach for qualitative data analysis should: 1) Determine products needed to achieve research and practice goals; 2) Decide a balance between the researcher's perspective and that of participants; 3) Evaluate time, staff, and resource constraints; 4) Establish the best mix of inductive and deductive procedures; 5) Ensure the best fit between the research purpose, audience, context, and judgment criteria (Ramanadhan, Revette, Lee, & Aveling, 2021).

Some considerations for research fit for this study were the purpose and nature of the research subjects: the study aimed to produce evidence that can be directly translated into practice to strengthen global health diplomacy and security, accelerate the promotion of health equity, and improve population health. Other pragmatic considerations were the availability of resources, the diversity of study participants and their perspectives, and the target audience for the study findings, which include current and future GHD actors and trainers.

As previously illustrated, this study design facilitates straightforward descriptions of participants' experiences and perceptions (Sandelowski, 2010), especially in areas where little is known about the topic under investigation (Glaser & Strauss, 2017). It also facilitates generating data that describe the 'who, what, and where of events or participants' experiences' from a subjective perspective (Kim, Sefcik, & Bradway, 2017). Thus, this design is also a responsive method to address pertinent global health issues, prioritizing the goal of contributing to change and quality improvement in GHD practice over furthering theoretical or conceptual understanding (Chafe, 2017) of existing knowledge, skills, and core competencies of GHD actors. Lastly, this design favors the presentation of research findings in a manner that directly reflects or closely resembles the research questions' terminology (Bradshaw, Atkinson, & Doody, 2017), as expressed earlier by the research aims and research questions.

II.   Data Collection

Sampling Strategy and Rationale

This research employed a purposive sampling strategy, using a mix of criterion sampling based on specific inclusion criteria and snowball sampling to allow for suitable referrals from interview participants. The purposive sampling technique is often used in qualitative research to "identify and select information-rich cases for the most effective use of limited resources" (Patton, 2015; Remler & Ryzin, 2015, p. 143). Criterion sampling facilitates the selection of 'rich' or 'excellent' examples of Global Health Diplomacy Actors to answer the research questions (Patton, 2015). This process required that the researcher engage in exploratory efforts to obtain existing information to identify and ascertain that interview participants meet the inclusion criteria. For example, when available, the researcher verified this information using participants' professional profiles (LinkedIn or X (formerly Twitter) to ensure they had the knowledge, experience, and expertise or background to respond to the research questions.

Additionally, the snowball sampling technique allowed interviewees to refer other potential study participants (Naderifar, Goli, & Ghaljaie, 2017), particularly within the Core and Multistakeholder categories that have greater specificity in their roles as GHD actors, and thus a relatively smaller GHD actor pool (See Figure 1). This sampling technique also gave the researcher access to participants that she would not have had access to otherwise. Thus, given the parameters of the study, including the efficiency of participant recruitment, data collection, and analysis, and the human resources available, this combined sampling strategy was implemented.

Inclusion Criteria

The inclusion criteria for the selection of GHD actors included individuals, representatives, or employees of government agencies, institutions, organizations, or entities that cultivate interactions and negotiations between and among each other and within and across governments and states, with the principal objective of improving population health. Based on the set forth aims, the researcher carefully selected study participants from the United States Core, Multistakeholder, and Informal Health Diplomacy categories. Inclusion criteria included English as a first language or fluent in English, employed/worked in the Global Health Diplomacy field for at least two years, specifically during the COVID-19 pandemic, and the participants' work was either US-based or US-focused, even if stationed in other countries. Those who did not meet these criteria were excluded from the study.

Recruitment Strategy

This study and procedures were reviewed by The George Washington University's Institutional Review Board (IRB), which granted the study "exempt status." The researcher reviewed open-source materials such as lists of global health or GHD conference delegates, documents, videos, publications, and social media platforms to identify credible GHD actors. Next, an Excel sheet of potential Core, Multistakeholder, and Informal GHD actors was created based on the aforementioned inclusion criteria. This document was shared with book committee members for participant recommendations and solicitation for participants' contact information (email addresses), where available. The researcher also leveraged personal networks and connections made at a local GHD training institute and some universities for suitable referrals.

The researcher contacted and invited potential Global Health Diplomacy actors via email or LinkedIn to participate in the study. The initial email or LinkedIn message [See Appendix 2] included an interview participation consent form [Appendix 4] and a research information leaflet [Appendix 5] with information similar in content to a consent form. The leaflet outlined the purpose of the research, operationalization of study concepts, research process, data collection methods, analysis, and storage. It also specified who will access the data, how it will be stored, for how long, and how the study findings will be utilized. In addition, the leaflet contained her contact information in case participants had questions or concerns about the interview process or needed additional details about the study. Once participants agreed to be interviewed, the researcher sent out a Zoom meeting invitation via the provided email with the agreed interview date and time. She contacted 71 people via email and LinkedIn; 32 responded, 11 declined or deferred to participate based on schedule conflicts, and 21 took part in the study:10 participants were male, and 11 were female.

Description and Administration of the Interview Guide

This study utilized in-depth interviews. This data collection method provided a structure that supports a systematic and comprehensive exploration of the questions and optimal use of the interview time (Remler & Ryzin, 2015, pg. 68). The Researcher chose this method as the most effective way to explore key informants' thoughts, perceptions, feelings, and beliefs about the knowledge, skills, and core competencies required for GHD practice.

Before commencing the interviews, she conducted two pilot interviews with respondents who mirrored the study participant pool. This process helped assess the cohesiveness and responsiveness of the interview guide to the research questions and identify potential flaws or limitations within the framing of the interview questions. While no major changes were made to the interview guide following the pilot interviews, the process helped underscore the importance of reiterating the definition of study domains as the questions were being posed to bring them to the forefront of the respondent's minds. The pilot interview also helped with reframing the definition of "core competencies to include the 'proper application of GHD knowledge, skills, and abilities at the right place and the right time.' The responses from the pilot interviews have been excluded from the study and were not analyzed.

The interview guide comprised five main sections: an introductory section, three content sections, and a final conclusion/reflection section. The following three sections comprised the main interview questions with corresponding prompts for an in-depth exploration of what participants thought were the skills, core competencies, and technical knowledge required for practicing global health diplomacy in a post-COVID era. Participants were asked to reflect on their personal experiences before and during the pandemic or from their general assessment of the GHD landscape and potential implications for practice in a post-COVID era. The researcher then asked the participants how they would define Global Health Diplomacy in a post-COVID era based on the information respondents had just shared. In the final section of the interview, the researcher asked participants if there was anything else about the research topic they wanted to add. This question was followed by a request for interviewee referrals and general interview close-out.

Study Procedures

The data collection occurred between December 1, 2023, and January 10, 2024. The researcher conducted the interviews via the Zoom platform, which has a feature that allows for the automatic generation of transcripts from audio recordings. The interview lengths ranged between 35 and 60 minutes. In total, the researcher conducted twenty-one (21) interviews: Core (7), Multistakeholder (7), and Informal (7).

Data Analysis

Qualitative data analysis requires organizing and interpreting raw data collected from participants' audio recordings, transcripts, and notes the researcher took during the interview process. She then followed the thematic data analysis procedure recommended by Braun & Clarke's six steps for systematic thematic analysis (Braun & Clarke, 2006), which are described in further detail in the 'Thematic Analysis' section below.

Data Preparation and Cleaning

After the interviews, the researcher retrieved the transcripts from Zoom, removed all personal identifiers, and renamed the transcript and their corresponding audio recording with a unique identification label. Each de-identified transcript was copied and pasted into a Microsoft (MS) Word document in preparation for cleaning, coding, and content analysis.

The transcripts and audio recordings were stored in separate cloud-based, password-protected folders. Only the folder with de-identified transcripts was shared with the research team to ensure participants' confidentiality and anonymity. As part of the data-cleaning process, the researcher reviewed each line of the transcripts while listening to the audio recording to ensure the transcription was error-free and any missed sections were filled in. This process also facilitated the generation of clean verbatim transcripts that captured all the participants' words, omitting false starts, filler words, repetitions, or requested redactions.

Data Organization and Reduction

The researcher used Dedoose qualitative software (Dedoose, n.d.) to organize and reduce the raw data to what was needed to answer the research questions. As a first step, the researcher developed a coding schema composed of a priori codes defined per the research domains in the interview guide. She created four main domains: 'GHD Knowledge,' 'GHD Skills,' 'GHD Competencies,' and 'GHD Definition' to facilitate sorting the data into these categories for thematic analysis. The researcher shared the coding schema with the Principal Investigator and book Committee Qualitative

Methods Lead for review and modification. Once the coding schema was approved, the researcher uploaded the de-identified MS Word transcripts into the Dedoose platform and entered the a priori codes.

Next, she sought to establish intercoder reliability using three interview transcripts, one from each GHD category. The deductive coding process helped reduce the volume of data by assigning specific words or phrases into the predetermined categories, as outlined by the coding schema. She and two research assistants read each transcript twice to familiarize themselves with the participants' accounts in response to the research questions before independently coding each one. All three reviewed each other's coded transcripts for coding similarities and differences. Coding dissimilarities were highlighted and discussed with the book committee chair, who acted as a mediator. Once a consensus was reached and intercoder reliability established, these codes were used to inform subsequent coding of the remaining transcripts according to the respective GHD categories.

The researcher began by doing open coding of the transcripts in Dedoose, using the constant comparative method (Glaser, 1965). Before generating a new code, she read the extract to see how well it fit into the initial coding frame, only generating a new code if the extract did not fit. The process was repeated, and the researcher refined the coding scheme through multiple rounds of coding as she built in new coding categories.

Thematic Analysis

The researcher followed Braun & Clarke's six steps for systematic thematic analysis to identify recurrent patterns of information generated through the coding process, which she organized to form themes and sub-themes (Braun & Clarke, 2006).

Thematic content analysis is the most common approach to analyzing exploratory, descriptive qualitative data by presenting the main elements of participants' responses or ideas (Green & Thorogood, 2018, pg. 258- 262). Thematic analysis also allows for systematically analyzing classified or coded data based on relevant themes or patterns. This process enabled the researcher to interpret the data by comparing or analyzing the association and relationship of individual themes within GHD actor groups and between groups. This type of analysis also facilitated the identification of and description of implicit (vague and unclear) and explicit (clear and unambiguous) ideas that emerged from the data (Alhojailan, 2012).

III.   Ethical Considerations

Institutional Review Board (IRB) Approval

IRB approval [FWA00005945] was granted on November 14, 2023, from the George Washington University Ethics Review Board [See Appendix 1]. Only after the review decision did the researcher begin interacting with study participants for data collection. The study was determined to be IRB-exempt as it poses no more than minimal risk to study participants (GWU Office of Human Research, n.d.).

Research Confidentiality

As noted above, after cleaning and de-identifying the transcripts, the researcher assigned each transcript a unique label to be used throughout the data coding and analysis process to maintain participants' anonymity and research confidentiality. All collected data was securely stored in a cloud-based, password-protected drive.

Informed Consent

Informed consent was sought and obtained from participants before the interviews. At the time of recruitment, the researcher shared study information, including data analysis and dissemination plan, with potential participants in plain language. The consent form also asked participants if their interviews could be recorded, allowing them to opt-out should they choose to. The researcher also let those who agreed to be recorded know that any identifying information will be excluded from the transcripts and that their responses will be confidential. Participants were informed that they could contact the researcher before the interview if they had any questions or concerns about the study leaflet or the consent form.

Consideration for Participants

While no participation incentives were given, the GHD actors agreed to participate in the study, understanding that they would be contributing towards potentially redefining and shaping the field of Global Health Diplomacy. Interviewees were informed that they could withdraw from the study at any time. They could also contact the researcher or Principal Investigator with additional questions or concerns about the study processes or data collection methods to ensure the study's appropriateness and validity. The study findings from the analyzed data will be presented in the next chapter.

Chapter Four: Results

This section presents a thematic analysis of study results in accordance with the study aims and corresponding research questions.

Study Participant Demographics

This study had twenty-one (21) participants. Of this number, 10 were male, and 11 were female. The Core, Multistakeholder (MSTK), and Informal (INFML) GHD actors had 7 respondents each. The table below presents study participants' demographic data according to GHD actor category and gender:

Table 6

Study Participant Demographics

GHD Actor	Gender	GHD Actor	Gender	GHD Actor	Gender
CORE 1	Male	MSTK 1	Female	INFML 1	Female
CORE 2	Male	MSTK 2	Male	INFML 2	Male
CORE 3	Male	MSTK 3	Female	INFML 3	Female
CORE 4	Female	MSTK 4	Female	INFML 4	Female
CORE 5	Female	MSTK 5	Male	INFML 5	Male
CORE 6	Male	MSTK 6	Male	INFML 6	Male
CORE 7	Female	MSTK 7	Female	INFML 7	Female

Research Question 1: What skills do GHD actors need for effective Global Health Diplomacy practice in a post-COVID era?

The results have been presented sequentially for each GHD actor category, beginning with the Core, Multistakeholder, and Informal categories. Global Health Diplomacy actors' skills have been distilled into six main thematic groups (with sub-themes), operationalized as follows:

1. **Interpersonal skills** collectively refer to traits and abilities that GHD actors expressed were critical for harmonious interactions with others from diverse cultural backgrounds to facilitate building and fostering relationships.

2. **Technical Skills** collectively refer to specialized expertise that GHD actors can leverage while practicing Global Health Diplomacy.

3. **Critical and Analytical Thinking** refers to GHD actors' ability to synthesize, analyze, and evaluate information in an objective and logical manner to make informed and sound decisions.

4. **Practical or Practice-Based Skills** refer to GHD actors' expression of practical skills employed in real-world GHD settings or Global Health Diplomacy skills in action.

5. **Learning** collectively refers to the process by which GHD actors acquire knowledge, information, or skills through a previous experience that leads to positive change that enhances practice.

6. **Communication skills** collectively refer to GHD actors' use of various communication formats, such as written, verbal, public speaking, elevator pitches, and crisis/risk communication, in GHD practice.

Global Health Diplomacy Skills Required by Core GHD Actors

This section presents the Core GHD actors' expressions of the skills required to practice Global Health Diplomacy. These skills have been grouped into the following categories: Interpersonal, Technical, Critical and Analytical, Practice or Practice-based, Learning, and Communication.

1. Interpersonal Skills

Interpersonal skills collectively refer to traits and abilities that Core GHD actors

expressed were critical for harmonious interactions with others from diverse cultural

backgrounds to facilitate building and fostering relationships. Core GHD participants

mentioned personal attributes such as empathy, humility, patience, flexibility, and active

listening as essential skills for diplomatic interactions. They also included other

interpersonal skills, such as the ability to see other stakeholders' priorities, perspectives,

equities, and motivations and being able to navigate these differences, especially when

they are in stark contrast to one's own:

> *"Diplomacy often requires quite a bit of patience, a tolerance for ambiguity, and willingness to compromise. I've seen a lot of people, and this is particularly the case with scientists, and I have to say frankly, you know, we send a lot of CDC doctors overseas and to these meetings. And you see the same thing sometimes, kind of with the military, where there's a right way and a wrong way. And you know the fact that sometimes you have to work with other systems and other perspectives, I think it is confounding for some people I know, over the years, we've had people whom we've sent overseas ended up having to get sent home because they ended up kind of offending the host country government"* (CORE 3).

The respondent further added:

> *"I think every country really has its own unique set of challenges. I think you sort of need to go into it with a real hard sense of the flexibility that you need to work in different systems"* (CORE 3).

Another Core GHD respondent likened diplomacy to "a contact sport" (CORE 5),

where actors needed to go beyond the exchange of emails and be physically present in the

same room as their counterparts to allow for face-to-face interactions, where "you are

jostling to get your point of view across" (CORE 5). They affirmed that diplomacy

requires patience while waiting for the opportunity to arise.

Core GHD respondents also highlighted the importance of cultural awareness and cultural humility in negotiations:

> *"A degree of cultural competency and humility go a long way. And when I say cultural competency, every country has a rich history and a rich culture that may or may not be understood or may or may not be known. But you have to be able to go into negotiations with one or multiple countries and have that in the back of your mind, knowing that the people that you are negotiating with have just as rich, just as complex, just as interesting a culture as you do. I'm not saying go in with rose-colored glasses because that is just as patronizing as going into a sitting like you know everything."* (CORE 5).

Demonstrating a "genuine interest in other people's cultures and environments" (CORE 6) was highlighted as a fundamental GHD skill. While this Core GHD actor said this ability did not require that Core GHD actors be "the world's most raging extrovert" (CORE 6), they had to be curious about what their counterparts were thinking, wondering, or needing. Another Core GHD actor asserted that having this skill also helps Global Health Diplomats pick up on subtleties, nuances, or non-verbal cues during exchanges:

> *"You have to listen to what's not being said, and I mention that because, for example, in Asia, especially if it's a big group, especially if leaders are at the podium, you're never going to hear 'no' or you might not hear an answer to a question either because they don't know. And it's face-saving, we use that in English all the time, and it is a very real thing in parts of Asia. Now, once the big meeting is over, you'll go down a quarter and hear them arguing furiously in a big room. Yes can mean yes; it can also mean maybe, and you will never hear 'no.' And so, you have to hear that, and you have to hear what questions they're not answering, and what topics they're not addressing"* (CORE 5).

One Core GHD actor noted the intricate link between cultural awareness and the ability to communicate more effectively vis-à-vis the intended audience:

> *"Some people think that, well, if I have a medical degree or a Ph.D. in virology or whatever, I must have everything I need to be a Global Health Diplomat. Actually, some of those people are really limited in what they can do because if they're only used to speaking in science or in medicine, they may lack the soft skills that you need to actually communicate with a wide audience. And that's really what you need to do in Global Health Diplomacy"* (CORE 6).

2. Technical Skills

This section presents the technical skills that Core GHD actors stated were important for GHD practice in a post-COVID era. Technical skills collectively refer to specialized expertise that GHD actors can leverage while practicing Global Health Diplomacy. There was some ambiguity around Core GHD actors' responses about the need for technical expertise, particularly with regard to having a solid clinical, scientific, or health background. Some felt it was crucial for building credibility and trust when dealing with other stakeholders, especially while working at embassies abroad, some of whom may or may not have scientific or technical expertise. Others said that although it held some advantages, it was not an absolute necessity. Participants' responses regarding the required technical skills are displayed in the table below.

Table 7

Core GHD Actors' Expression of Required Technical Skills for GHD Practice

Technical Skills	Core GHD Actor Excerpt
Project Management	*"A good sense of program management is helpful. It's not necessarily so helpful in the actual sitting around the table, hashing out a text, or being a diplomat. But in terms of working with the big multilateral organizations in terms of saying, okay, we need to look at your program. We need to look at your budget. We need to see your strategic plan. It's now 2023. We need to understand where you are getting at in 2024, and it helps to have some degree of experience in running a project. So, you can understand what's feasible and what's important, and that builds your diplomatic portfolio"* (CORE 6). *"I think the Global Health Diplomacy world really does need people with some program management experience. I think that's something that's actually quite lacking, and the ability to manage a budget, not so much the ability, the experience of having managed a budget and a program and seen it through over a multi-year period. A six-month stint is not enough. But you know, really being able to go through several cycles and understand the complexity"* (CORE 3).
Logistics and Supply Chain	*"I used to say that every functional supply chain system is functional in the same way, and every dysfunctional one is dysfunctional in a different way. And I think every country has its own unique set of challenges. In a pandemic response, a lot of what*

	you really need is logistics experience and a very basic understanding of supply chains. I've never been a supply chain expert, but I've often worked on the margins of it. But I really am taken with just the complexity of that world, and not just the complexity, the difficulty of it" (CORE 3).
Financial Resource Management and Utilization	*"An understanding of economics and finance is something that I think would be very helpful because, increasingly, much of what is being discussed in the diplomatic space has to do with funding. And it has to do with where the resources are coming from and how are they being used?"* (CORE 6).
Data Analysis and Statistics	*"I think it's also important to have strong skills in scientific communication, being able to take that data and translate it into digestible, actionable nuggets for the public that will be attractive and clicked on"* (CORE 2). *"So, in terms of specific skills that might be useful, the ability to understand data statistics, all those sorts of things"* (CORE 6).
Epidemiology and Disease Transmission	*"I think it's important to have skills in epidemiology, scientific communication, and biostatistics to understand and interpret the massive amount of data associated with our disease surveillance systems, understanding where the gaps are and knowledge, and being able to target them"* (CORE 2). *"We certainly need skills of understanding the basics of epidemiology. We need to be literate in questions about how disease is spread, what are the threats, what are our behavioral characteristics, where we can, perhaps, minimize our chances of being infected, and whether the actual characteristics of the virus or the pathogen itself, that would that we need to be aware of and how those play out"* (CORE 1).
Health or Scientific Expertise	*"I think the number one thing that you need is to be a health expert of some kind; you need to know biomedicine; you need to understand zoonotic diseases… you need to basically know what happens to a human being and the environment"* (CORE 4). *"So, I think that being an expert in health or science generates a lot of trust. You're not seen as a diplomat; you're seen as a subject matter expert. So, when you are dealing with a foreign country, either because you work at an embassy or you work from Washington on health security issues, they will trust your knowledge and your reputation as an expert and not your reputation as a diplomat who is seen as pursuing other interests other than human health"* (CORE 4). *"Having experience as a clinician, on some level, as a physician, as a nurse, as a pharmacist gives you a lot of insights. It gives you a lot of credibility. When you deal with various players, it helps you immediately. You have this kind of basic knowledge about the way that a health system functions, the way that a facility works, how a clinician speaks to a patient, and then what the implications are of that for all the other things you're looking at in the system"* (CORE 7).

Broad Mix of Technical Expertise	*"I think the clinical one is really a very strong one. I think it's incredibly helpful, but also having a real technical background in things like supply chain and logistics or having worked in regulation"* (CORE 7). *"If you participated in clinical trials around drugs, you have a much better understanding of what it takes to fast-track a medical countermeasure. You understand how to communicate risk when you're talking to politicians"* (CORE 7).
Non-Health/ Non-Scientific Expertise	*"Many of the world's really accomplished Global Health Diplomats have no technical training whatsoever. They are lawyers or political scientists. If you do have some degree of technical background, it doesn't necessarily need to be in the biomedical life sciences. It can be in informatics. It can be in engineering. It can be in logistics, as long as you've got those core attributes of being curious, being something of a self-starter, and being interested in other people"* (CORE 6).
Generalist	*"Another thing you need to be able to do is to acknowledge that you're a generalist and say 'I will get back to you' if you don't know the answer to something and figure out which experts you need in the room to inform decisions and acknowledge they don't necessarily have to come from all fields. You cannot have all of the same voices at the table; otherwise, it's an echo chamber. So, you need a diversity of voices for representation, but also because you make better decisions. And I would argue that the same applies to health diplomacy, health security, and all of it"* (CORE 5).

3. Critical and Analytical Thinking Skills

This section presents CORE GHD actors' ability to synthesize, analyze, and evaluate information in an objective and logical manner to make informed and sound decisions. A senior Core GHD Actor shared an experience about balancing risk and uncertainty in the US response to the AIDS epidemic:

"AIDS was really not a fast-breaking outbreak; this was something we've developed for many years, and by the time it became a priority agenda in Africa, we knew a lot about the virus, and, in fact, by the time PEPFAR started we had the countermeasure. There was a lot of uncertainty about whether it would work in the way we hoped in African surroundings and whether there would be long-term consequences that would have a political push back on the US. Because we didn't know the long-term consequences of this very toxic drug, and we were giving it not just to a few people in the experimental state but to tens of thousands of people all at once. So, there was some uncertainty, and then there was a lack of

*evidence about the prevention of AIDS. So, that was an example of where you
really need to weigh the evidence that you could find in journal articles. Did this
apply here? Could we deal with the risk, uncertainty, and lack of evidence?"*
(CORE 1).

4. Practical or Practice-Based Skills

This section presents the practical skills that Core GHD actors stated were
important for GHD practice in a post-COVID era. Practical or practice-based skills refer
to GHD actors' expression of practical skills employed in real-world GHD settings or
Global Health Diplomacy skills in action. Core GHD actors referenced diplomacy as a
critical skill for GHD practice, noting its relevance for generalists and specialists as an
underlying principle guiding personal and professional interactions and health
negotiations.

One Core GHD actor affirmed:

> *"If you wanna talk about global health diplomacy or health diplomacy, you must
> also understand diplomacy. [It's in] the word itself. You need to be diplomatic in
> the way you communicate things, the way you hear things and the way you treat
> people. You need to understand that, although you are a scientist or a biomedical
> professional of some kind, sometimes, when you are confronted with a pandemic
> or a health security crisis, there are many other things at play that are not just the
> pure basic science or the fact"* (CORE 4).

Another Core GHD actor relayed that being a generalist facilitated diplomatic
interactions, and GHD practitioners could rely on their team members for specific
technical skills as needed:

> *"I think, in general, diplomacy skills often benefit from a generalist approach.
> And these are often different skill sets. I mean, you don't need a lot of supply
> chain experts who are also good generalists. So, you really need a team
> approach. But yeah, often the people who seem to do best in this world are people
> who are generalists who get the diplomacy"* (CORE 3).

One Core GHD actor noted that in real-world scenarios, practicing diplomacy was not without challenges, especially when dealing with multiple perspectives or representing views one may not necessarily agree with:

> *"The other thing is as a diplomat, your job is also to represent the views of your country, and you need to be able to do that sincerely without taking offense. Sometimes, you might have to represent ideas you don't agree with, and you have to figure out how to do that in a way that you feel preserves your personal dignity, but you can truthfully represent those ideas. That's a hard thing to do"* (CORE 5).

According to one Core GHD actor, diplomacy also requires a delicate balance of knowing when to be persuasive or prescriptive whilst interacting with policymakers. They further added that the process requires knowledge of existing norms within countries and how these can be applied in other countries:

> *"The skill of diplomacy is really finding areas of agreement and convergence and exploiting them and minimizing areas of divergence. So that takes skill, both listening and being able to understand the position of the actor across the table"* (CORE 2).

Practical or Real-World Global Health Diplomacy Experience

Core GHD actors stated that practical experience in Global Health Diplomacy is critical to bilateral and multilateral discussions about global health funding or foreign assistance. One Core GHD actor explained that some GHD actors' theoretical understanding of global health concepts often did not reflect the real world and failed to consider "how things can go wrong" (CORE 3).

> *"Most of the problems that we have when we're in Geneva and talking about Global Health Diplomacy are that there really are rifts between developed and developing countries, and I think it's not a bifurcated world anymore. It's really more of a trifurcated world now, where a billion people are living in low-income countries. But then you've got about 5 billion people living in these middle-income countries who have an array of challenges. They, in some ways, look like rich countries, and in some ways, they look like low-income countries, and a lot of*

people live in between. And I think that complexity is really where a lot of our biggest challenges are" (CORE 3).

Another Core GHD actor affirmed that in real-world scenarios, global health issues are not isolated from other ongoing or developing crises. They explained that scenarios like forced migrations, conflict, ethnic tensions, political reasons, or scientific or biological considerations might explain why global health programs fail:

> *"In my experience, diplomacy really is important to advance public health goals. And there's, of course, the whole other side of it that we're increasingly discovering that it can be, although it's not used as much as it could be, a way of improving political or economic relations between countries. But it can be a common interest of countries, even where the political relations may be fraught"* (CORE 1).

Multisectorality in Diplomacy

One Core GHD actor divulged that as a critical component of their diplomatic function, GHD actors need to understand how the role and responsibilities of a Global Health Diplomat cut across multiple sectors:

> *"I think there should be this inherent acceptance of multisectorality. An ambassador, for instance, is responsible for political, economic, management, and counseling. In other words, the well-being of citizens and public diplomacy, as well as questions of long-term and short-term relations, are where you have to both manage crises and look at long-term policy interests. You have to look at the interests of your headquarters and the interests of the country where you're working; all of these have public health implications. But often, biomedical people or people working on development programs don't have that broad perspective. And so, it seems to me that health diplomacy is a valuable input into public health work. Most of the people who come in response to an outbreak or have been working their whole lives on the biomedical responses to an outbreak don't have the political, economic, or supply chain logistical, even sociological, ethical questions that ambassadors have to deal with in all sorts of responses"* (CORE 1).

Understanding the Intersection between Health and Foreign Policy

One Core GHD respondent stated that for GHD actors to be effective, they must understand the intersection between health and foreign policy objectives and how to represent their country's foreign policy priorities:

> *"You need to understand that you are not just a scientist when you are in one of these positions, that you have a policy role to play, a global policy role to play, an international policy role, that you're representing an ambassador and a mission abroad, and it's not just the science. There's a lot on how you communicate things, how you prioritize the interest of your own country, the country that you're representing, the interest of the host country, so you can concile and reconcile, and have agreement on very contentious things. So, you have to be a negotiator. You have to be a good communicator"* (CORE 4).

One Core GHD actor stated the need for GHD actors to understand how various governments talk or interact with each other, how to craft messages, and how to approach or utilize diplomatic communication channels for formal demarches or complaints. They further added that GHD actors need to understand how specific global health objectives within a program interlock with those of the host country government's goals and figure out where those points of intersection are:

> *"For Core diplomats that represent the government to another government, it's really important to understand what are the goals of that government in our country? What are they trying to do? Even on a smaller scale, understanding how to look up the foreign policy objectives in every country. So, you can go on the web and look up what the US government is doing in Ethiopia. What are the goals? We're an open society. Informal actors like those in academics, the general public, people in the NGOs, or multistakeholders like the WHO, World Bank, the IMF, and UNICEF, could look up the Integrated Country Strategy of the US Government in any country, and then figure out how their goals interdigitate with the US Goals and find those areas of confluence or divergence. So, [knowing] this is not routine; unless someone shows you this, people aren't going to understand that we do have this very open, transparent, accountable process to the American people."* (CORE 2).

Global Health Diplomacy Training

Core GHD actors also highlighted the need for training within the field of Global

Health Diplomacy; one Core GHD participant called for better leverage of skills that

diverse GHD actors already possess instead of seeking out new training:

> *"How do we use the respective skills that diplomats, biomedical people, or health policy people already have to work together to advance or address some of the challenges or problems we already have? I think we should make sure that diplomats all have a basic statistics course, or all have a basic epidemiology course; [it] wouldn't be a bad thing. But I would be reluctant to go down that track. I think diplomats have to learn a lot about many things they haven't had college courses in"* (CORE 1).

5. Learning

Learning collectively refers to the process by which GHD actors acquire

knowledge, information, or skills through a previous experience that leads to positive

change that enhances practice. In this section, Core GHD actors expounded on the

process through which GHD actors promptly acquire knowledge, information, or skills

through previous experience and decision-making as new data emerges.

Access to Timely Information

Core GHD participants stated that finding credible information in a timely manner

is critical for diplomats in general and Core GHD actors in particular. These actors

mentioned that they often rely on prior experience and personal judgment when dealing

with information sources and, to some degree, trial and error to ascertain which

information sources are reliable and to what extent.

According to one Core GHD actor, this was one of those make-or-break skills for Global

Health Diplomats:

> *"I think for diplomats, one of the key questions is where do we look for information? To whom do we reach out? And how do we evaluate that information in the context of policy [considering] the science is never perfect? In*

*the case of COVID-19, we actually got it wrong for a long time, and it's
something that should have been much easier for scientists to determine." (CORE
1).*

Using a real-life example, the Core GHD respondent went further to share some

considerations that factored into the diplomat's decision-making process, which they said

were not necessarily unique to GHD:

> *"They [diplomats] have to do it on the fly. You have to have just-in-time
> information about a tremendous number of subjects and sort of figure out who
> you trust, who has that information, and how you put that information in the
> context of what other uses of this are. [For example] what are the risks of giving
> the Ugandan army, which has huge human rights problems, this [night goggles]
> technology? Could it be misused? Is it going to be controlled? Is this actually fit
> for purpose? And all these questions that you have to ask using other kinds of
> experiences you have as a diplomat. It's not unique to health or unique to military
> assistance or unique to, you know, trade issues"* (CORE 1).

Similarly, another Core GHD actor discussed the importance of maintaining diplomatic

channels through which diplomats can send and receive information in real-time. They

reflected on how shutting these channels impeded their ability and function at the heart of

the pandemic:

> *"Prior to COVID and before the previous [US] administration, we had over 50
> [communication channels]. I think there were more than a hundred different
> bilateral mechanisms by which we communicated with [country redacted]. It's a
> really great way for us, as a government, to get insights into what is a very closed
> society and how it functions in a broader range of academic disciplines, from
> economics to political to biomedical. And we shut that down as a government so
> that basically shut off our ability to get insights. All that was left were these
> informal channels between individual diplomats. Without the formal channels,
> you really have a hard time mobilizing the government to have leaders meet and
> have concrete discussions with real outcomes that will advance our
> interests. Without the ability to advance our interests in a formal channel, our
> ability to function would be hampered. So, you had all of these diplomats and
> public health professionals who had all of the competencies and skills necessary
> to advance, but the system itself didn't work. The whole system really lacked the
> ability to make concrete adjustments, concrete agreements, and outcomes"*
> (CORE 2).

Informed Decision-making Using New or Emerging Data

One Core GHD participant emphasized the need for diplomats to evaluate the information they already have and emerging data to make decisions. While this respondent recognized that many decisions are made amidst uncertainty, as diplomats may not have all the information to paint a complete picture, they cautioned against decision paralysis:

> *"Both scientists and diplomats tend to have thinking patterns that look at previous experiences, that look at models that both are open to changing the way you do business but also resistant to that. And so, I think looking at both of those ways of thinking and approaching problems is a key to health diplomacy; you need to appreciate the scientific use of evidence and the sense that more research needs to be done"* (CORE 1).

The respondent further added that diplomats needed the ability to make decisions even when they did not have a complete understanding of pressing challenges:

> *"There's a lot of uncertainty and a lot of assumptions here, and diplomats need to take action. Now, you can't just wait until all these uncertainties are resolved or more research needs to be done. You actually have to do something, and you have to weigh these risks. And so, I think diplomats are relatively good at, if they have the proper information, trying to figure out which uncertainties mean that we actually shouldn't move ahead quickly and which ones mean that we can manage the risks that are here, and if we need to change course to do that"* (CORE 1).

6. Communication Skills

Core GHD Actors underscored the importance of gaining mastery of various communication formats and the ability to synthesize information, making it easily digestible and comprehensible for the intended audience. They also needed to know who to rally around the discussion table to ensure they had a balanced assessment and alternative perspectives when evaluating situations for which there are far-reaching consequences.

> *"Communication skills! Communication skills! Communication skills! They need to be able to write, synthesize information from different places, and communicate*

ideas, but they also need to be able to listen to both what is said and what is not said, and they need to know how to ask the big-picture questions. They also need to know who to look to for answers and not assume they have all of them. Sometimes, they need to know how to bring different actors into a room who need to talk to each other. But you need to create some people say negative space, I say, safe space where it's nobody's turf. So, they all have to talk to each other, and they can contribute to something" (CORE 5).

The same GHD actor also explained some challenges when writing for particular

audiences and the need to consider the lenses through which their writing might be

scrutinized:

"And it's really hard to write for government because, you know, everything we do in government is couched in ifs, ands, or buts. There's a lot of passive, aggressive language in government. Still, because I have to use it, and I think I'm a pretty good writer, I think some of my writing has gotten worse because of this passive, aggressive language that its surrounded in. And you understand why? Because you have to couch things like, well, we could do this, or we might be able to execute this because there are people who are looking and going, 'Oh, she said, 15 billion dollars! Where did she get that figure from?'" (CORE 5).

Another Core GHD actor illustrated how information can be communicated to avoid

overwhelming the listener or decision-maker, emphasizing the need to ensure the main

points are not lost in the broader narrative:

"It really, really helps to have really great communication skills. Verbal communication, written communication, the ability to make presentations, the ability to collapse complicated issues down into their elements to say, okay, here are nine important things we need to bear in mind. They're all important. Five are urgent; these two drive everything else. So, we need to, above all else, address the two. The two will help us master the five, and then we'll have the luxury to deal with everything else." (CORE 6).

Some Core GHD actors also accentuated the skill to communicate scientific or technical

information to non-scientific or non-technical counterparts, stakeholders, or the wider

public, who may often find it challenging to understand, synthesize, or interpret scientific

data:

"A lot of times, I am talking to people who know nothing about health, who don't actually care about health, but they know it's important to them politically, and I

need to synthesize information. They don't want to know about the 35 studies that have something about transgenic mice and cancer; they could care less. Now, my friends at NIH care about those 35 studies and then factor in all that. But I need to figure out what the bullet point is from that so that I can say in clear, intelligent language that doesn't talk down to anyone about what the point is and so that leader can either make a policy decision or convey the message" (CORE 5).

Similarly, while recognizing the value of being skilled at communicating, one respondent went further to say that Core GHD actors or diplomats first needed to know how and where to access information and how to make those communication channels more useful. Another Core GHD actor described some ways in which public and private communication may elucidate or obscure the messaging during global health events:

"Sometimes, when you are confronted with a pandemic or a health security crisis, many other things are at play that are not just pure basic science or fact. And I think that we've seen with the infodemics in the last pandemic, it's how you communicate; it's not enough to tell people that this is the science, this is a molecule, or whatever. You really need to understand communications and what you do at large in terms of risk communication and private communication. It has to be the way you communicate with your colleagues from other countries, from international organizations about the things, and the motives behind things" (CORE 4).

Knowledge and Mastery of Foreign Languages

Some Core GHD respondents asserted the importance of understanding and speaking a foreign language, which they said served as a gateway into the host culture and facilitated cross-cultural interactions and understanding of the actual meaning of certain words, phrases, or generally what is being said or not said:

"One thing that has been very important for me is to know the host country's language. If you are in a post in a foreign country, I mean it's super essential. Unless you are in an English-speaking country, it's very difficult to communicate if you are not fluent in the language. I mean, it's not impossible, but if you want to have in-depth diplomatic relationships and technical relationships, you need to be able to catch the subtle things in the conversations. I sometimes see with my colleagues that we leave meetings, and they are like, 'they said yes to everything, that's great!', and I say, no, they did not" (CORE 4).

Another Core GHD actor added that while having a foreign language may not be necessary to function in some locations, it helps the GHD actor understand the host government's messaging to its own people:

> *"It helps understand how the government communicates its messages to its domestic population, and those insights were incredibly valuable to the United States Foreign Policy agenda. So, this was a time when the public health questions rose directly to the top of the government, and that doesn't always happen"* (CORE 2).

The Role of the Media and Social Media on Population Behavior

One Core GHD respondent stationed abroad at the time of the pandemic discussed media outlets' distinct role in public health messaging and shaping public opinion, using the events of the pandemic within the US as a comparative point of reference:

> *"For a break from my work, I would just watch the news and try to understand what was happening. Normally, domestic news dominates 90% of news broadcasts. As COVID progressed, international news suddenly started growing, especially US news. Normally, maybe 5% of the news would be international, and a little bit would be about the United States. That became about 30% of the news on what was happening in the United States. They were doing it for a very specific reason: to juxtapose their society with the United States and assure their people that look, this is a society in total chaos. It really reinforced their messages to calm their population and provide competent leadership in their own messaging to their people"* (CORE 2).

The same Core GHD actor also highlighted the influence of social media on people's behavior and called for GHD actors and the public health community to play a more active role in promoting evidence-based health messaging. They also underscored that GHD actors know how to utilize social media platforms:

> *"I think in this information age; it's exceptionally important to understand how social media influences people's behavior and the skills necessary for not just navigating through the various social media platforms that people use but really curating these messages and participating in the dialogue. Often, scientists will ignore the cacophony of chaos that surrounds that. But there's real truth there. I think it's one of the purest forms of our 'public square,' and as public health professionals and scientists, having the skills to be able to use those tools, to be able to advance public health messages is super important"* (CORE 2).

Global Health Diplomacy Skills Required by Multistakeholder GHD Actors

This section presents Multistakeholder GHD actors' expression of Global Health Diplomacy skills required for Global Health Diplomacy practice. These skills have been grouped into the following categories: Interpersonal, Technical, Critical and Analytical, Practical or Practice-based, Learning, and Communication.

1. **Interpersonal Skills**

Interpersonal skills collectively refer to traits and abilities that GHD actors expressed were critical for harmonious interactions with others from diverse cultural backgrounds to facilitate building and fostering relationships. Amongst the Multistakeholder GHD actors, the phrases "having soft skills" or "people skills" (MSTK 5) were mentioned with specific examples of personal attributes like empathy, emotional intelligence, cultural intelligence, compassion, honesty, and trustworthiness as integral to relationship-building. One Multistakeholder GHD respondent stated that relationships were the anchor of all diplomatic interactions:

> *"If you are not in a relationship with the people across the table from you, you can come and do stuff, spend your money, gather data, and take it where you came from; all of those things can be possible. But quite frankly, if there isn't a partnership between you and the folks across the table for whom this relationship is supposed to be beneficial, I think that you are not leveraging diplomacy because the backbone of diplomacy is that it is about relationships. They could be good, they could be bad, but you are in a relationship with each other"* (MSTK 1).

Some Multistakeholder GHD respondents emphasized that a key first step to building any relationship is understanding the people or populations one might be interacting with, their positionality, and the contexts and locations in which these interactions occur. They affirmed that this ability requires GHD actors to "see things from a different perspective"

(MSTK 6) and seek to understand the "cultural factors that cause people to do what they do" (MSTK 4) as they attempt to advance alternative solutions.

One Multistakeholder GHD actor stated:

> *"I'm more and more amazed with how different [it is] when you have CDC talking to USAID or NIH talking to the Bill of Melinda Gates Foundation. Never mind the US talking to China or Kenya, just how different institutions have their own cultures. And when I say pandemic treaty, someone else is thinking of something totally different and just the incredible cultural difference. Even within the same US Government, two agencies will think of things and do things entirely differently. So, just learning about those kinds of cultures in a very broad sense, not just sort of traditional national cultures, but institutional cultures, and learning how to learn about that and work in those different environments, I think, is especially important (MSTK 5).*

Another Multistakeholder GHD actor said leveraging Global Health Diplomacy was a means of navigating challenging bilateral relationships to achieve desirable health outcomes by finding creative avenues of engagement:

> *"For example, we had this complicated relationship with [Country redacted] about the types of [diplomatic] exchanges because [Country redacted] is in some category of x, y, and z by our government. The health program became the vehicle through which the relationship was being advanced. So, in [Country redacted], we can't give them government-to-government financing, for example, but we are able to do a lot of things in a more diverse way with our partners. And so, we exercise our health diplomacy in a different way"* (MSTK 1).

Another Multistakeholder GHD actor mentioned that GHD actors must not be "bogged down into certain beliefs" (MSTK 6) based on their own previous experiences but keep an open mind as they interact cross-culturally. One Multistakeholder GHD actor also recounted their experience of how they sought to foster mutual understanding between their team and international passengers at a US port of entry at the height of the pandemic:

> *"You did have to come from a place of understanding. When we had to speak to passengers and explain to them, 'Hey, you have a positive COVID test; you can't travel,' and that was hard for passengers. Some of them were going to family reunions. Some of them hadn't seen their family since the borders were closed.*

Some of them had a lot of different things that they were going through, that they weren't taking into consideration that, 'hey, I can't fly,' and us telling them they can't fly. They didn't understand the connection between, 'Hey, we're trying to prevent this spread of COVID, and that's why we're recommending that you don't continue your travel.' They couldn't wrap their heads around that. So, it was really an important aspect for us to come from a place of understanding and understanding their anger wasn't directed towards us. It was really just because they were going through so much, and we're throwing this negative information at them" (MSTK 4).

Multistakeholder GHD actors relayed that relationships also depend on establishing trust and credibility between interacting parties, especially amidst the growing mistrust of policymakers within the United States:

"And so, to say, oh, I'm a diplomat, like, what does that mean? It means that I'm engaging and creating a relationship so we can have some sort of data exchange later, or you'll tell me about an outbreak. So, the CDC, for example, has people who've been in the country for many years, like, say, a country in Africa that has a PEPFAR program. They've had an office with people, not the same people, over time many different people in that office for more than 20 years. So, the government in that country knows CDC from like, 'oh, they help us with these outbreaks.' They help us with HIV, they help us with tuberculosis, whatever. And so, there's trust there. And because of that trust, there's a diplomatic relationship" (MSTK 7).

Another Multistakeholder GHD actor shared some personal attributes they thought made some people do better than others in the practice of Global Health Diplomacy:

"It probably has a lot to do with a certain level of comfort and discomfort with unexpected things and a certain amount of humility because we all have a lot to learn. All the attributes of people who are good at working in teams, collaboration and communication, trust, transparency, and being evidence-based. No one person, or group or institution can do everything, so I think all the attributes of people who are good at working in teams and collaboration are essential" (MSTK 7).

Another participant within this group shared a similar sentiment about the importance of collaboration and teamwork when working with other partners during the COVID-19 response. For yet another Multistakeholder GHD actor, with the pandemic came the realization of more similarities than differences between high-income and low-income countries or financial aid donors and aid recipients, who were facing the same issue at the same time:

> *"So we would go places and would even talk about bringing models from our own CDC, or we're bringing models from how community programs are run in the United States, and then we get confronted with a pandemic, and it's the first time that I realized that we are no different from the people we were helping to serve because we also had denials of science. We had our own version of witchcraft; we called it conspiracy theories. And so COVID, for me, was a great equalizer in actually making that relationship that I'm describing happen on a more even playing field. Because our superiority would come because we had a lot of technical knowledge, and we had a lot of money. It turned out we were just like all the other humans, and that humility is something I am constantly reminding myself of"* (MSTK 1).

2. **Technical Skills**

Technical skills collectively refer to specialized expertise that GHD actors can leverage while practicing Global Health Diplomacy. Among the Multistakeholder GHD actors, there was a stronger emphasis on the need for technical expertise for GHD practice in a post-COVID era, particularly in global health, public health, or other health-related areas. Multistakeholder GHD actors asserted that being perceived as a 'content expert' was crucial for establishing legitimacy in multistakeholder interactions with foreign counterparts and during negotiations of technical intricacies such as vaccines or drug trials. These respondents within this category also highlighted the importance of data sharing and knowing how to use computers. These Multistakeholder GHD actors' technical skills have been summarized and presented below in Table 8, which captures the required technical skills, including research, knowing how to conduct technical negotiations, and understanding why data and resource sharing are critical in emergency responses:

Table 8

Multistakeholder GHD Actors' Expression of Technical Skills Required for GHD Practice

Technical Skills	Multistakeholder GHD Actor Excerpt
Research	*"Do your research and also take assessments of the skill sets that you may not be strong in. I'm not a big researcher, so I'm taking additional courses on those things that I know I'm weak on in terms of analyzing technical research and understanding the strengths of those research studies.? We've been taught to connect the dots if you will, and you can't connect the dots if you have no idea what the dot means, right?"* (MSTK 2).
Computer Skills	*"[You need] informatics skills"* (MSTK 5).
Technical Negotiations	*"So, if you negotiate at a technical level, making sure that you understand that certain processes take time in terms of the trials and things you're negotiating or the feasibility of saying, we'll do this in 3 months while you know that technically, that is not possible, but you do want to agree on something because that will help you access samples from countries or countries will find the best possible place for them to be analyzed. The ability to understand the short and long-term benefits of a negotiation. It's not a health, medical, or technical skill. It's a very different kind of skill. Also, understanding the global health instruments and laws and treaties and all of these things that are out there to situate your discussion in that context and also anything else that was negotiated before you"* (MSTK 6).
Public Health or Global Health Expertise	*"Quite frankly, I work in an environment where there are a lot of generalists. Just today, I was commenting on the fact that you know we needed a coordinator in South Africa, and people were like, well, could we just get a foreign service officer? And I was like, there are definitely some parts of health diplomacy that anyone can do as a diplomat, but this is embedded in some knowledge about health and health topics, not just in a superficial way, but where you are actually contributing substantive knowledge. So, no health diplomat without some health training, knowledge, experience to offer, because anybody can be the gatekeeper to exchanging facts from one side to the other"* (MSTK 1). *"You have the types that come to it with a very strong technical public health background, but then they add some other skills to it. They may or may not be completely perfect because all their experience is based on that health topic. If they were thrown to negotiating Arctic security, they may pick up some other skills they can then apply in health, but they don't have that chance because that's not what they do. They only do this when they have to. If you are trained in health, it's the ability to take things to a different level. And if you're not trained in health, I guess a better understanding of certain health aspects is important"* (MSTK 6).
Understanding Implications for Data, Knowledge, and Resource Sharing	*"I think COVID also made us realize how small the world really is, how connected it really is. And so, issues of data sharing, whether that's numbers of cases or sequences of variants or just general*

	information, sharing and transparency, really was highly problematic during COVID. And [it was], therefore, recognized as a really important global good to share data and then also to share knowledge, like a policy. So, I think all of that is in today's global health world, critical pieces that might not have totally been there before COVID" (MSTK 7).
Technical Expertise or Background	*"You can't just show up and assume, well, because I'm from this Northern institution, I have something to give, not necessarily! What's your competency? What do you bring to the table that isn't already here? So often that's very technical, like epidemiology training, or something, [whether] it's HIV, or it's TB, or it's malaria, or it's laboratories, or it's outbreak investigations, where you bring to the table a certain skill set that is desirable. And through that relationship, you create trust, and that trust is really the diplomacy. So, I feel [that] to be a Global Health Diplomat, it's important that you have a content area"* (MSTK 7). *"I guess, really having a basic understanding of some of the more biomedical and clinical and epidemiological aspects of diseases and health and the statistics and transmission, and just having a kind of a basic health literacy--global health literacy."* (MSTK 5). *"Understanding global health governance and who the key actors are, the role of nation-states, the World Health Organization, others like Gavi and the Global Fund and those governance and financing aspects. Another would be around the law and policy environment, the International Health Regulations, and the Pandemic Treaty that's being worked on, and more explicitly, how some of these countries negotiate and come up with agreements. And what the role is of countries or how they can try to control the flow of people and goods, how the issues around sample sharing and those legal policy aspects. I guess also have some familiarity with the research. And you know how medical countermeasures are developed, and the manufacturing and supply chain issues around that would be important"* (MSTK 5).
Flexibility in Resource Allocation and Utilization	*"So, I think some of the things coming to mind are really having flexibility, how you're programming funds, and then how you're giving them to partners to be able to use those funds. That was something that, in the COVID pandemic, we weren't able to do as best we would have liked to because the funds either weren't available. We had to wait until they were disbursed and available to be sent to partners. That was really a challenge. So pre-positioning funds so that they're readily available and that's also related to stockpile supplies"* (MSTK 3).
Financial Management and Accountability	*"I worked a lot on the supply chains during COVID with PEPFAR, and the other point that comes to my mind is organization, especially when you're working with donor funds, especially when you're working with US taxpayer dollars. You need to do a lot of record-keeping, and making sure you're really organized is critically important because you're going to have to report on the effectiveness of the use of those funds and where they went"* (MSTK 3).

3. **Critical and Analytical Thinking Skills**

Critical and analytical thinking refers to GHD actors' ability to synthesize, analyze, and evaluate information in an objective and logical manner to make informed and sound decisions. Multistakeholder GHD actors highlighted the importance of situational and contextual understanding by considering the political, economic, sociological, legal, environmental, and other factors that may be at play as they practice in GHD. One Multistakeholder GHD actor underscored the need to be better prepared for potential arguments against one's proposition or plan of action. Another respondent within this group highlighted the need for GHD actors to understand the changing global health landscape and to critically reassess the global health partnerships in a post-COVID era to ensure more equitable health outcomes:

> *"Post-COVID, the big thing that has come up that global health actors are thinking about more than they did before COVID (although I don't think it has anything per se to do with COVID) is the whole landscape of diversity and equity and global colonialism. I think that the idea that the European or Western or North American institutions are not the answer and that there are really important leading institutions in the Global South, if you will, and that recognition of their value and their contribution, their partnership is really an important and newer area of global health that I think wasn't there before. What it means is the way that we work with institutions and individuals has really changed, or should change, to be the right global health partner"* (MSTK 7).

4. **Practical or Practice-Based Skills**

This section presents Multistakeholder GHD actors' expression of required practical skills employed in real-world Global Health Diplomacy settings.

Practical or Real-World Global Health Diplomacy Experience

Multistakeholder GHD actor respondents also expressed the importance of GHD actors gaining real-world or practical experience while actively working in the field of GHD, preferably across a variety of non-health sectors:

> *"We invented the term Global Health Diplomacy, but there are a lot of diplomats
> who are stationed, or who are generally doing this day in and out, not just for
> health, but for other things. For them, it doesn't really make a huge difference"*
> (MSTK 6).

Other Multistakeholder GHD actors shared a similar perspective, recommending that

GHD actors gain practical experience whether they were generalists working at

embassies, research, or public health institutions. One Multistakeholder GHD actor noted

Global Health Diplomacy in practice was often the exchange of scientific information

and resources for solving health issues:

> *"So, when you think about what it means to be a Global Health Diplomat? It's not
> really about diplomacy in and of itself to me; it's really about a relationship that
> creates a diplomatic channel, a working relationship where you bring value"*
> *(MSTK 7).*

Global Health Diplomacy Training

A few Multistakeholder GHD respondents discussed the relevance of GHD

training, especially in key concepts like global health security, which they felt GHD

practitioners and policymakers were yet to grasp in the post-COVID era. One

Multistakeholder GHD actor talked about learners' approaches to global health and

Global Health Diplomacy, cautioning against substituting one for the other:

> *"I do teach Global Health Diplomacy, and I catch myself repeating to the
> learners that they are not there to learn about global health. So, I think it's
> important not to mix the fact that it is in this interdisciplinary area, but by no
> means are you going to learn about everything in global health in such a course.
> So, if you want to learn about global health, take another course"* (MSTK 6).

Individual and Institutional Adaptability, Flexibility, and Risk-Taking

For one Multistakeholder GHD actor, one of the benefits that emerged from the

pandemic was that it helped upend the status quo, allowing individuals and organizations

to explore creative ways of working and making them more inclined to take risks:

"I also saw a lot of younger staff put in important positions, getting a chance to demonstrate their abilities and then going on to other roles. So, I really saw COVID advance a lot of people's [in development] careers because they were able to pivot, find new jobs, and take risks" (MSTK 3).

Negotiation Skills

About half of the Multistakeholder GHD respondents in this category mentioned negotiation as a critical GHD skill that diplomats were required to have, independent of whether they were negotiating for health-related outcomes or others such as agriculture or cease-fires. Multistakeholder GHD actor said negotiations were always happening 'day in, day out' in line with disease outbreaks or other emerging global threats. They did, however, share some important considerations when approaching negotiations:

"I think the skills also will vary from place to place. I think it depends on who the negotiator is or who is responsible and what their worldview, training, or work experience has been. If you are looking globally, which countries are involved, which players are involved, and culturally, other things will come into play, such as negotiators, being male or female. Being from certain parts of society, a million things come into play. For negotiation skills, understanding stakeholders and different kinds of players and the ability to realize the need for an outcome, setting priorities for your negotiation, and understanding who you're negotiating on behalf of; what are the red lines, or what are the expectations from that negotiation" (MSTK 6).

Leadership Skills

One Multistakeholder GHD actor acknowledged the importance of leadership, describing it as an ability that is honed through practice over time:

"I think leadership [is important] as well; it's something that people develop over time. But the most effective teams that I've been on have really charismatic leaders that are adaptive and have those qualities that people want to follow them, want to be on their team, and [be] engaged" (MSTK 3).

Understanding the Role of Public Health

One Multistakeholder GHD actor recognized how public health permeates every aspect of life and called for GHD actors to better understand the role of public health at the individual and population levels. They also stated the importance of making sure the

public health sector and public health initiatives received the funding they deserved:

> *"We need to advertise [public health], but we need to put the resources there. We need public health, but technology has not even caught up with the public health departments; they have antiquated equipment, and they were faxing. A lot of folks look at public health as though it's only for folks like the marginalized populations and those who are at the lowest socioeconomic rungs. But we found in COVID that public health is for everyone" (MSTK 2).*

5. **Learning**

This section presents Multistakeholder GHD actors' expressions of the process

through which GHD actors acquire knowledge, information, or skills through a previous

experience that leads to positive change that enhances practice. Multistakeholder GHD

actors highlighted the importance of GHD actors' ability to promptly access information

as well as knowing how to manage misinformation and disinformation.

Access to Timely Information

Reflecting on the events of the pandemic, one Multistakeholder GHD actor

commented on the need for GHD actors to know how to access and utilize credible

information in emergencies:

> *"Being able to find information, especially with COVID, where there weren't textbooks on SARSCoV2 because it didn't exist. So, just learning how do you actually keep up to date and get information? How do you determine and detect credible information versus misinformation versus disinformation? So that would be an important skill – learning, finding, and using information"* (MSTK 5).

Managing Misinformation and Disinformation

A few Multistakeholder actors highlighted the learning opportunity the pandemic

offered GHD actors around mis-and-disinformation and discrediting of public health,

considering several public health practitioners had been caught off-guard:

"I think there was a very crucial lesson learned about the pandemic because for all my years in global health, all of the understanding, sometimes the privilege, whatever it was, the tools that I had to come to that table…until something happened that suddenly was happening to us at the same time as it was happening to the partner countries that we had been collaborating with, we never actually questioned ourselves. So, all of a sudden, we were home here in America, watching the public reject public health. We'd never thought about that" (MSTK 1).

Another Multistakeholder GHD actor mentioned the need for GHD actors to

understand the roles and functions of the US Government's Legislative, Executive, and

Judicial arms:

"Something that they don't teach in medical school that I had to learn in the US context is how Congress actually works. For example, what are the implications of an Executive Order? What is PEPFAR, or what is the difference between the actual authorization between an Executive Order and the commission of PEPFAR? So, just learning how to be an effective Global Health Diplomat in the US context, especially within the existing framework of US Federal Government institutions, is important" (MSTK 5).

6. **Communication Skills**

Communication skills collectively refer to GHD actors' use of various

communication formats, such as written, verbal, public speaking, elevator pitches, and

crisis/risk communication, in GHD practice. Across the Multistakeholder GHD category,

the art of communication spanned several domains, taking into consideration the context,

location, purpose, and target audience. For one Multistakeholder GHD actor,

communication during the negotiation process was relational and required clarity,

authenticity, and self-confidence:

"I think communication can be broadly defined, both in terms of how you relate in the process and how you relate with other members of your own team or your capital; these contexts are very diverse. I think communication is an extremely important skill here. It's also how you communicate with your other stakeholders because, at the end of the day, the Global Health Diplomat may have many competing priorities thrown at them. But how they clearly communicate why

certain things may have to be done a certain way, that has to be done very carefully" (MSTK 6).

Another Multistakeholder GHD actor stressed that the role of the communicator was just as important as the audience, as whatever message was being communicated would vary depending on whether the information was publicly facing or for whom it was destined:

> *"I always tell folks when they go in for a meeting or a briefing, it's not about you; you know the information. The information isn't for you; you're trying to convince someone to use and apply the information. So, you have to do your research and understand your audience to know what their skill sets are. If you're talking to a bunch of technical researchers, then that's great; stay in the technical realm. But suppose you're talking to a mixture of both allied health scientists as well as health care administrators and educators. In that case, you have to understand how to articulate in their language the research you're trying to convey or whatever it is you're trying to get them to do"* (MSTK 2).

Another Multistakeholder GHD actor added:

> *"Learning how to speak and write for different audiences, learning about all the different communications channels, from scientific publications to the site formerly known as Twitter, what kinds of information or arguments you need to use for different audiences. Knowing all the communications, I think, is an important skill"* (MSTK 5).

Knowledge and Mastery of Foreign Languages

Multistakeholder GHD actors mentioned that GHD actors' understanding and mastery of foreign languages is a critical skill. These Multistakeholder GHD actors asserted that this ability allows for informal understanding and discussion amongst stakeholders or partners who may not speak English or for whom it may not be a first language, avoiding a communication breakdown:

> *"Knowledge of [foreign]languages is also extremely important. The main language of communication is English because a lot of international organizations operate that way, but regional communications and negotiations do not happen in English. Sometimes, negotiations take place through translation, and the quality, level of understanding of that translation, and use of appropriate translation become extremely important. Having more than one language at your disposal is extremely important. It allows you to break the ice with your potential partners in negotiation and understand the nuance of certain expressions or a*

*certain array of situations where a straight translation may not deliver that
aspect. Obviously, a diplomat who speaks languages is always better than a
diplomat who doesn't speak the languages; there's no question about that"*
(MSTK 6).

For another Multistakeholder GHD actor, being able to learn and speak a foreign became

a defining moment in how they were able to do their job:

*"We had a lot of international passengers; we worked at a quarantine station at a
port of entry during the pandemic and eventually came to a point where we were
screening a lot of passengers from Spanish-speaking countries, and we only had
one Spanish speaker. So, I spoke with that Spanish-speaking colleague and was
like, 'listen, you need to teach me Spanish.' Specifically, I had that colleague
teaching me how to say whatever questions we had to ask the passengers, proper
pronunciation, and everything. We were trying to ask for certain documentation
to do our job, trying to communicate and help educate some of these passengers,
but we couldn't if we didn't speak the language. I think this is the most important
skill in Global Health Diplomacy because you can have all the information in the
world and communicate till you're blue in the face, but if you're not speaking the
same way, you're not going to get your message across"* (MSTK 4).

Global Health Diplomacy Skills Required by Informal GHD Actors

This section presents Informal GHD actors' expressions of skills required for

Global Health Diplomacy practice. These skills have been grouped into the following

categories: Interpersonal, Technical, Critical and Analytical, Practice or Practice-based,

Learning, and Communication.

1. **Interpersonal Skills**

Interpersonal skills collectively refer to traits and abilities that GHD actors

expressed were critical for harmonious interactions with others from diverse cultural

backgrounds to facilitate building and fostering relationships. Amongst Informal GHD

actors, these skills include a range of personal abilities and characteristics such as

empathy, emotional intelligence, and self-reflection, which are integral to forging

connections with people from different backgrounds:

> *"Emotional intelligence, and the ability to connect with others across cultures, across nationalities. It is a skill that I don't know if it can be taught. But I mean, certainly, you can rely on translators, but being able to develop relationships, I mean, all of this depends on mutual collegial relationships"* (INFML 3).

For one Informal GHD actor, cultural awareness goes beyond personal interactions to include political settings as well:

> *"Having an understanding of language and culture, understanding more than one language is helpful, I think. Having an understanding of the political cultures that exist where everyone is willing to work is critically important"* (INFML 5).

Informal GHD actors also mentioned other relevant skills for practice, including servant leadership and collaboration, especially in emergency settings. They said:

> *"Being a servant leader, one that really is there to ensure that they can support one another in the implementation of a project, and it doesn't matter who gets recognition for the idea. I would add optimism because there's so much uncertainty. And you're not entirely sure if the idea is gonna work, if there's going to be continued funding. You're also bombarded with seeing the devastation that's happening around you, so you need to have leadership that has optimism that we can pull through this and can convey that to your stakeholders"* (INFML 7).

The same respondent also mentioned the ability to network and develop collaborative partnerships for successful project implementation and outcomes by leveraging existing systems and resources to avoid duplication of efforts.

2. Technical Skills

Technical skills collectively refer to specialized expertise that GHD actors can leverage while practicing Global Health Diplomacy. Informal GHD actors' perspectives of the technical skills required for post-COVID GHD practice were relatively diverse. The table below presents GHD actors' expressions of skills in specific technical areas such as One Health and systems-thinking, clinical expertise, program management, data analysis and statistics, and knowing how to steward financial resources, which they stated were integral to GHD practice:

Table 9

Informal GHD Actors' Expression of Required Technical Skills for GHD Practice

Technical Skills	Informal GHD Actor Excerpt
One Health and Understanding of Systems Thinking	*"I think anybody moving forward has to be very familiar with the One Health concept. For me, One Health is the concept that human, animal, plant, environmental, and ecosystem health are linked: that's my working definition. [One Health] is absolutely instrumental to use as a framework moving forward because when we're talking about global health, we can't just focus on humans; we don't live in a vacuum"* (INFML 3). *"And then systems-thinking, which kind of ties into the public health ethics, emergency preparedness, and One Health, because I feel like One Health really pulls in all of the areas of public health that could lead to a potential disaster or emergency. Both naturally, man-made, or otherwise"* (INFML 4).
Project Management	*"I would say program management is really, really key; making sure that we're looking at a work plan, [that] we're flexible with what activities we all want to do as stakeholders, but we're referring to that as to what our goals are and making sure everybody's aligned with those targets"* (INFML 7).
Clinical Expertise or Healthcare Background	*"It would be great for them [GHD actors] to have some healthcare background; they don't have to be healthcare providers, but having some knowledge of the global healthcare landscape that they maintain at all times is really important"* (INFML 1).
Data Analysis and Statistics	*"You do need to know data [analysis] really well. Everybody has to be comfortable with looking at trends, looking at caseloads, and referring to data to make decisions"* (INFML 7).
Financial Management and Utilization	*"Having financial wherewithal to understand your position in the organization you work for and their financial resources as it applies post-COVID because we found that during the pandemic, many people didn't even understand their financial resources and their limitations"* (INFML 1).

3. Critical and Analytical Thinking Skills

Critical and analytical thinking refers to GHD actors' ability to synthesize, analyze, and evaluate information in an objective and logical manner to make informed and sound decisions. Informal GHD actors mentioned contextual and situational understanding as a critical skill for GHD practice. They stressed that GHD actors need to be aware of the cultural, economic, and political contexts in which they operate, locally

and nationally. Informal GHD actors also emphasized the need for GHD actors to

understand the country's capacity to prevent, detect, and respond to local health events to

prevent them from spreading across regions or borders:

> *"Ask yourself 'how did the country perform during the COVID era, what was its response, and what was its capacity?' I think engaging in Global Health Diplomacy should also take into account what has been done with that particular country or region in terms of pandemic preparedness and the amount of resources that have been brought into bear. What are some of the capacities that have been developed? If there are any assessments that might have been done by the WHO, like a Joint External Evaluation or something like that, that needs to be taken into account. Some of the joint external evaluations that are done post-pandemic are even more important to see what their scores might have been compared to the ones before and after COVID, whether you see an increase or decreasing scores, and what specific capacities are performing and at what level?"* (INFML 6).

Another Informal GHD actor called for the need to assess the successes and failures of

the COVID-19 response to adequately inform training domains for GHD actors in a post-

COVID era.

4. Practical or Practice-Based Skills

This section presents Informal GHD actors' expression of required practical skills

employed in real-world Global Health Diplomacy settings. Informal GHD actors

highlighted the need for GHD actors to have real-world experience in pandemic

preparedness and response efforts, negotiation, and the ability to identify and engage

various key stakeholders, amongst others. They also proposed training domains for GHD

actors.

Knowledge of Stakeholders and Multisectoral Engagement

Informal GHD actors underscored the need for GHD actors' knowledge of key

stakeholders, their roles and objectives, and how to engage as being critical for successful coordination and collaboration amongst NGOs to maximize available resources and avoid

duplicating interventions:

> *"We need to know what they are communicating and what particular aspects of pandemic preparedness they might be working on with the country. Coordination and collaboration with the stakeholders are important so that we don't sort of tread over one another. We should be more or less synchronous rather than actually being competitive and trying to cut each other, which a lot of NGOs, unfortunately, and even other organizations, tend to do. So, I think it needs to be a joint, collaborative, coordinated effort with the Government"* (INFML 6).

Another Informal GHD actor acknowledged the need for GHD actors to be adept at

intentionally collaborating with other stakeholders across non-health sectors for more

robust policy and programmatic outcomes.

> *"We're really pushing hard for political scientists, economists, public policy individuals, and public admin people to be more engaged in global health. They're not, but we need them. I mean, I'm a physician, but I need them as much as, hopefully, they need us"* (INFML 5).

Individual and Institutional Adaptability, Flexibility, and Risk-Taking

Informal GHD actors also cited adaptability, flexibility, and the ability to take

risks at the individual and institutional level as essential skills for GHD actors, especially

in emergency scenarios where resources need to be rapidly mobilized to save lives. One

Informal GHD actor recounted:

> *"There was flexibility in our line items on how to spend our money. As you know, certain funding mechanisms, especially USG, are very strict about taking money from one line item to the next, which doesn't allow for creativity. You constantly have to go back to your donor and wait for a response, and you can't move fast on implementing the project. You can't do that [in emergencies]; you need to be able to take action and move forward. That flexibility from [Donor name redacted] was really helpful, allowing us to be creative. When there was a decrease in the COVID caseload, there were patients with long COVID who also have noncommunicable diseases like diabetes and hypertension. We were able to address those issues amongst these patients as well"* (INFML 7).

Negotiation Skills

One Informal GHD actor mentioned the importance of knowing how to negotiate as a foundational skill for Global Health Diplomacy. They added that being a good negotiator requires making concessions where possible, knowing one may not always get all they want out of a negotiation. However, the same Informal GHD actor cautioned that GHD actors should ideally not walk away from the negotiating table empty-handed either:

> *"Part of negotiating is learning people aren't always nice. You can try to be as respectful as you can be. But sometimes you have to take the gloves off because other people are taking the gloves off so that you can negotiate for what you need for your particular country or whomever you are representing. I think, in a post-COVID era, you really have to take into consideration"* (INFML 1).

Pandemic/Emergency Preparedness and Response

About half of the Informal GHD actors highlighted the importance of GHD actors building their skills in pandemic preparedness and response, considering the likelihood of future pandemics:

> *"The countries that had to deal with SARS in 2003 actually fared better than those that did not because they had practice. You get better at things. Well, the US dodged the SARS bullet in 2003, and while that was good, it meant we didn't get practice, so we got hammered with COVID"* (INFML 3).

Sharing their concerns about emerging health threats, an Informal GHD actor talked about the challenges the planet faces due to climatic variations that pose tangible threats to global health security, sustainable agriculture, and food security.

> *"The Biological Weapons Convention doesn't have enforcement capabilities. It's been weakened, the norms have been ignored, and we're entering dangerous territory with [a] lack of trust between countries. At the same time, we've got almost 8 billion humans on the planet, and they have to be fed in a sustainable way. Agriculture is the foundation of civilization; climate change threatens agriculture, and agriculture threatens climate change. About a third of the greenhouse gases, the most potent ones, methane, and nitrous oxide, come from agriculture. So, we've got serious issues confronting us that people in global*

health security must recognize and be able to discuss with their counterparts in other countries" (INFML 3).

Understanding US Foreign Policy Works and its Impact on Global Health

One Informal GHD actor discussed the intersection between US Foreign Policy and Global Health. They alluded to a 'primary tension' between the global health community's approach to addressing health issues versus that of foreign policymakers. The same respondent also mentioned the need for GHD actors to seek to understand the political agenda-setting process, as well as the role of foreign policymakers:

> *"Foreign policymakers have to do triage. It's a ruthless process of setting priorities with limited resources. Foreign policymakers determine what happens in diplomacy; the global health community doesn't do that. So, you're getting this bigger and bigger gap between the problems foreign policymakers have to identify, deal with, and then they send the diplomats out to do stuff and this sort of ever-expanding global health claims that everything is interdependent and interlinked, and therefore we need to handle sort of everything all at once, everywhere"* (INFML 2).

The same Informal GHD actor further disclosed that the post-COVID was going to be driven by even more 'ruthless' priority setting by foreign policymakers, with each country striving to protect its own interests:

> *"And here is where the skills are going to differ, based on what a country's foreign policy interests are. So, is the United States gonna focus on PEPFAR or pandemic preparedness? The idea that there are synergies between these things, in my experience, is largely a fantasy. Particularly in this world, the competencies and skills that I need are to advance or protect my country's interests, not save lives globally; it didn't operate that way before. So, there is still a need, I think, for skills and competencies and understanding of how foreign policy is made within a country, and that every country is struggling with that now because of geopolitics. It, unfortunately, warps how we think about every issue. Even issues like health, where if we take action, it isn't going to produce any geopolitical benefits, even if we argue that it's going to"* (INFML 2).

Understanding the GHD Landscape

One Informal GHD actor called for an understanding of the current Global Health

Diplomacy landscape, taking into account the challenges, changes, and ongoing

geopolitical tensions that becloud bilateral and multilateral discussions and interactions:

> *"When we first started talking about health diplomacy or Global Health Diplomacy, nobody knew what you were talking about because it was never an important foreign policy issue. So, the sky was the limit, and that was also a case where you had political space to do that where there wasn't geopolitics. It was a unipolar system, and that unipolarity, where the hegemon is a liberal democracy, opened up political space for civil society institutes, not just in the US but in Africa. With the return of geopolitics, the role of non-state actors has shrunk enormously. It isn't what it used to be, right? We no longer talk about Bill Gates as sort of being another great power. Rockefeller is now doing climate change. I don't have to tell you about problems in the United States, right? There's no consensus on healthcare, there's no consensus on public health, there's no consensus on how to deal with pandemics, there's no consensus on climate change. Again, that's different; that's changed, except on climate change, we never had our act together on that. So, I don't know what skills I need because who am I interacting with, and on what issues?"* (INFML 2).

The same respondent asserted that the skills GHD actors need will ultimately be defined

by their countries' present and future foreign policy priorities, which will also inform

global health funding. This Informal GHD actor went further to challenge the assumption

that GHD practice was geared towards improving population health. They asserted that

while this has been a key objective in the past, newer geopolitical priority changes within

the GHD actor pool and a rise in authoritarianism dominate current political discussions

and negotiations, raising the question of whether global health is of prime concern:

> *"The decline of democracy worldwide means that the political space for civil society, even companies, and non-state actors, is truncated for reasons that have nothing to do with global health. And again, it's not just the global health problem; for example, you have authoritarian countries shutting down human rights organizations around the world. Their space isn't there anymore. There is no Chinese Bill Gates. There's no Chinese Rockefeller, and the same is true on the Russian side, too. So, it's slanted in a way that seems to have this idea of how we used to do it because the US and other Western democracies were the engine of global health activity. And it's leaving out what I always considered part of health*

diplomacy, which was that I'm using health to get something else, and there is disagreement about whether or not these issues are important anymore" (INFML 2).

The respondent maintained that in this modern era of GHD, actors must first seek to understand these changes and their government's objectives and then draw from skills they already have or develop new required skills for adeptly navigating these issues:

> *"I think plug-and-play skills are going to be important. I don't necessarily know what I need to do to handle this issue; where do I go to find that expertise? It's hard to say what those skills are a priori until I have my political instructions from the White House, the National Security Council, the State Department, USAID, the CDC, or whoever it might be. Once I know what I'm supposed to do, once I know how much money I have, then I organize the skill set for that"* (INFML 2).

Global Health Diplomacy Training

When reflecting on GHD training areas, one Informal GHD actor suggested leveraging the One Health matrix as a framework for training GHD actors, considering how critical it was to GHD practice in a post-COVID era:

> *"Using it [the One Health Matrix] at the satellite level linking food safety security, anti-microbial resistance, and emerging diseases with climate change. And it's all linked to fecal production. Interestingly enough, we're producing a lot of fecal waste and not talking about it. So, we're generally focused on the front end, but we've gotta look at the back end, too; that's part of Global Health Diplomacy. We're drowning in our waste, not only plastic but fecal as well. And that fecal waste is contaminating soils and waters in the atmosphere and everything else"* (INFML 3).

For another Informal GHD actor, Global Health Diplomacy ought to be a core part of global health training, considering most people who have a biomedical background have not been expressly trained in these skills:

> *"I hope that more individuals who are global health practitioners will actually acquire the skills of Global Health Diplomacy. Because if you're interested in impact versus performance, then you have to learn and understand the skills that are going to be in your book, I'm sure. And we in global health should be humble enough to understand that we have to acquire those skills. Since most people in global health come from a biomedical background, it's not our training.*

But it's essential that if we want to have an impact that we have some of these skills. So, I hope that Global Health Diplomacy becomes a core part of global health training" (INFML 5).

Understanding Political and Power Dynamics

Some Informal GHD actors emphasized the need for GHD actors to understand political and power dynamics. They further explained how political will and power dynamics between and within countries impact global health outcomes:

"I think they [GHD actors] need to understand the dynamics of politics and the dynamics of power. They need to understand and be sensitive to the incentives and motives of power structures at international, national, and subnational levels and between countries. Each one is unique, every permutation, every combination of what I mentioned is a unique relationship, and people need to understand that" (INFML 5).

Similarly, another Informal GHD actor underscored how crucial it is for GHD actors to have a clear understanding of these power structures, the role of global health actors and decision-makers within these structures, and their commitment to global health or lack thereof:

"The other thing is also taking into account the country commitment itself is also important, as well as the global commitment towards that country, and also some of the global organizations like WHO as well as some of the other regional partners, whether they are governmental or non-governmental partners to support that particular aspect. So, in Global Health Diplomacy, you also have to take into account the level of receptivity. From the policymakers in terms of the changes that they need to make because a lot of countries are very proud of their own country and their ability to do things themselves, but at the same point in time, how do you balance that in a diplomatic way, and communicate that to the policymakers and to the responders or to line ministries within a government to be able to deal with that" (INFML 6).

Understanding Public Health Ethics and Ethical Implications

One of the Informal GHD actor respondents noted the lack of consideration of the ethical implications of public health practice in future emergencies, particularly in the absence of a clearly defined code of public health ethics:

"In public health, we've often utilized medical ethics to potentially the detriment of our field. Because we are very unique, there are different considerations that we as public health practitioners, especially Global Health Diplomacy practitioners, need to take into consideration. Without a predefined code of ethics that is specific to that [public health], there are a lot of situations that could potentially happen that would be unethical" (INFML 4).

5. Learning

This section presents Informal GHD actors' expression of the process through which GHD actors acquire knowledge, information, or skills through a previous experience that leads to positive change that enhances practice. Knowing how to manage infodemics was highlighted as critical for GHD actors, especially in a post-COVID era.

Managing Misinformation and Disinformation

One Informal GHD actor described being overwhelmed and astounded by the amount of misinformation and disinformation that surfaced with the COVID-19 pandemic:

"Being prepared for the politicization of public health was something I don't believe any public health official was prepared for, even though we had gone through a pandemic previously, it wasn't to this level, and the pushback was not to this level. I don't think we were prepared for the impact of social media on this information and misinformation related to vaccines. So, I really think that actors have to really be engaged with their communities just to keep their finger on the pulse" (INFML 1).

6. Communication Skills

Communication skills collectively refer to GHD actors' use of various communication formats, such as written, verbal, public speaking, elevator pitches, and crisis or risk communication, in GHD practice. Communication was a salient theme amongst Informal GHD actors, with respondents in this category emphasizing GHD actors' ability to communicate with diverse stakeholders to facilitate proper dissemination of information, especially during emergencies. One respondent stated that the ability to communicate provides a "good foundation" (INFML 1) for diplomatic interactions:

> *"It's about how you communicate effectively across multiple different stakeholders and avenues throughout an emergency in order to make effective policy decisions and communications out to the population"* (INFML 4).

Another Informal GHD actor mentioned how the ability to deliver a clear PowerPoint presentation helped fast-track their donors' funding decisions during the pandemic, as opposed to going through the traditional grantmaking process:

> *"Something that was very, very unique with our project; typically, an RFA [Request for Application] or RFP [Request for Proposal] comes out, you write and wait to hear back. In an emergency, you don't have time to do all that. So, what we did was they gave us the opportunity to do a PowerPoint presentation. It's just easier. It distills all the information helps, and you make a decision really quick"* (INFML 7).

This previous section presented a thematic analysis of the Core, Multistakeholder, and Informal GHD actors' responses to the required skills for GHD practice. The following section will focus on GHD actors' responses to the core competencies necessary for GHD practice.

Research Question 2: What Core Competencies do GHD actors need for effective Global Health Diplomacy practice in a post-COVID era?

Core competencies collectively refer to the essential knowledge, skills, and abilities that GHD actors need for Global Health Diplomacy and the proper application of these knowledge, skills, and abilities by GHD actors at the right place and time to practice Global Health Diplomacy effectively. The results have been presented sequentially for each GHD actor category, beginning with the Core, Multistakeholder, and Informal categories. Global Health Diplomacy actors' skills have been distilled into six main thematic groups (with sub-themes), operationalized as follows:

1. **Interpersonal Competencies** collectively refer to traits and abilities that GHD actors expressed were critical for harmonious interactions with others from diverse cultural backgrounds to facilitate the building and fostering relationships.

2. **Technical Competencies** collectively refer to specialized expertise that GHD actors can leverage while practicing Global Health Diplomacy.

3. **Critical and Analytical Thinking Competencies** refer to GHD actors' ability to synthesize, analyze, and evaluate information in an objective and logical manner to make informed and sound decisions.

4. **Practical or Practice-Based Competencies** refer to GHD actors' expression of practical skills employed in real-world GHD settings or Global Health Diplomacy skills in action.

5. **Learning Competencies** collectively refer to the processes by which GHD actors acquire knowledge, information, skills, or abilities through a previous experience that leads to positive change to enhance GHD practice.

6. **Communication competencies** collectively refer to GHD actors' use of various communication formats, such as written and verbal communication, public speaking, elevator pitches, and crisis/risk communication, in GHD practice.

Core Global Health Diplomacy Actors' Core Competencies

This section presents the expression of core competencies required for Global Health Diplomacy practice by Core GHD actors. While the Core GHD actors did not mention any interpersonal core competencies, findings from the other themes are presented below.

1. **Technical Competencies**

Technical competencies collectively refer to specialized expertise that GHD actors can leverage while practicing Global Health Diplomacy. This section presents Core GHD actors' expression of required core competencies for Global Health Diplomacy practice in a post-COVID era. In the table below, respondents underscored the importance of having some knowledge or background in medicine or science to understand the intricacies behind pharmaceutical discoveries. They also mentioned that it was crucial to adequately manage donor funding and navigate the challenges of global and local supply chains.

Table 10

Core GHD Actors' Expression of Required Technical Competencies for GHD Practice

Technical Area	CORE GHD Actor Excerpt
Financial Knowledge, Stewardship & Accountability	*"How did you spend money that was already appropriated? You had a program; how did you spend that money wisely, avoid or minimize the risk, maximize the benefit to the people, and do no harm?" (CORE 1)*
Technical Expertise or Technical Background	*"In terms of the scientific skills, one of the things that I've discovered here in Geneva is that an astonishing number of diplomats really don't understand how science or medicine works. They don't understand what a clinical trial is; they don't understand the phases of getting a drug approved. They don't understand the financing. We've been doing a lot of the Pandemic Accord negotiations here in Geneva. Even amongst some really well-trained diplomats, you realize they actually don't know the technical issues behind how surveillance works, epidemiology, the intrinsic qualities of the diagnostic tests, and then there are the characteristics of the population, and you need to have both; otherwise, you're not going to get useful information. So, some degree of training in this is how science works or this is how responding to an outbreak works" (CORE 6).*
Logistics and Supply Chain	*"Understanding the realities of trying to manage a complicated logistics supply chain when you don't have reliable power, when you don't have good communications, and so forth" (CORE 6).*

Government Culture vs NGO Culture	*"There's the difference between government culture and NGO culture, those sorts of things. Some familiarity with the field experience of delivering health and healthcare is probably pretty useful, I think"* (CORE 6).

2. Critical and Analytical Thinking Competencies

Critical and analytical thinking competencies refer to GHD actors' ability to synthesize, analyze, and evaluate information in an objective and logical manner to make informed and sound decisions. Core GHD actors relayed that in addition to knowing where to find credible information sources, GHD actors also needed to know how to assess the quality of information that would ultimately guide their ability to make rational decisions:

> *"To me, the most important is that you have to be able to know and have a good deal of confidence in how you deal with sources of information. And what do you rely on there? And that's mostly through experience or a little trial and error. Ebola was also a little bit different in that you were dealing with denial and how did you get countries that didn't want to admit that they had a problem or that they couldn't deal with it to figure out what partners they needed or what that changes they needed in their own approach to deal with their own population, which had huge potential to spread beyond their own borders? They weren't looking at it from that point of view at all, and we're trying to minimize the problem or saying that they could deal with it, and so these require a different set of skills, a different set of partners, but it is an analysis of the situation"* (CORE 1).

3. Practical or Practice-Based Competencies

This section presents Core GHD actors' expression of practical competencies applied in real-world GHD settings or Global Health Diplomacy competencies in action. Core GHD actor respondents emphasized the underpinnings of diplomatic engagements, determining and setting priorities, and the need for training in specific GHD domains as some of the essential areas for GHD practice.

Diplomacy

All the respondents in this Core GHD actor category expressed that diplomacy is integral to the GHD practice and the role of GHD actors. Some Core GHD actors regarded 'diplomacy or traditional diplomacy' as encompassing health and non-health-related discussions, negotiations, or interactions with other counterparts, versus Global Health Diplomacy or Health Diplomacy, which they said was specific to health-related interactions or outcomes. For one Core GHD actor, traditional diplomatic skills provide the baseline for interpersonal interactions and which GHD actors can learn to be more proficient practitioners:

> *"There's the traditional diplomatic skills, which are some understanding of rhetoric, persuasive speaking, some training on how to write a decent memo, to be brutally honest, how to actually put together a good PowerPoint presentation, some of this is salesmanship, right? It's how to get your point across in 2 or 3 minutes, how to present yourself, how to be engaging; and we all think we know how to do this, but we can all probably learn to do it better. I certainly could learn to do it better. Speaking, in terms of allocution skills and, as I said, soft rhetorical skills"* (CORE 6).

The respondent went further to highlight the importance of practicing negotiation and mediation in more egalitarian settings where the dynamic between parties was not overshadowed by one party's dominance over the other, as can be seen in financial donor-recipient relationships:

> *"When you're representing the world's biggest donor, it's not a true bilateral relationship. The power dynamic is really offset. So, you don't necessarily learn the skills the right way because you're basically representing a massively disproportionate amount of influence in the room. So, learning from that would be helpful. It might be helpful to do externships, honestly, with some smaller, highly influential but less wealthy, less domineering countries, and the Europeans are often sometimes rather good at this. After all, they've had to learn to play because they represent countries with smaller populations, smaller economies, but generally a highly developed diplomatic sense. They've learned how to use the soft skills of mediation and accommodation and triangulating between positions"* (CORE 6).

Agendas and Priority-Setting

When reflecting on agenda and priority-setting, one Core GHD actor mentioned

that although setting an agenda can lay the foundation for negotiations, GHD actors need

to be savvy in identifying what topics were immediate diplomatic priorities versus those

that were not:

> *"Diplomats put our priorities on to other people's agendas, so some of the skills
> are the determining what's a priority. What the timing is of interventions. The
> sense of 'is this important, and is this the right time to take up a public health
> issue.' There are trillions of public health issues we should be dealing with, but
> not all of them deserve to be diplomatic priorities now or would be successful as a
> priority. So, it is a question of timing and priority setting"* (CORE 1).

Collaboration and Cooperation

When discussing this sub-theme, Core Global Health Diplomacy actors

emphasized the importance of regional and international collaboration and cooperation as

a means of strengthening global health security and containing the spread of infectious

disease outbreaks. One Core GHD actor said:

> *"I think, hopefully, everyone saw how important this is; in neighboring countries,
> whatever happened in one country happened in the other, and you had to have all
> those provisions for what you're gonna do. For example, Mexico was the first
> country that we donated vaccines to, even before President Biden announced the
> global donation campaign. Why? Because we're so intertwined, our supplies are
> interdependent, our food and medical supplies are interdependent, and our
> defense supplies are interdependent* (CORE 4).

Another Core GHD actor shared how diplomats were instrumental in rallying

governmental and non-governmental partners to champion and advance global health

priorities:

> *"I think that diplomats have some skills that can advance public health goals. And
> therefore, certainly implies that this is something that's done around the world
> between nations in which governments and partnerships between governments
> play a role. Also, those relationships in foreign countries, for instance, the US
> Government, would entail partnerships, not just with governments, but with other
> players with whom diplomats and embassies would come in contact"* (CORE 1).

The same respondent went further to share a comparative perspective of bilateral

collaboration during the Zika outbreak and the early days of the COVID-19 pandemic,

noting some of the barriers to sample sharing at critical moments:

> *"Zika, I put in a different category; there, you needed some kind of political framework for scientists to cooperate. We had things that could help the Brazilians. They were doing things that could help us, except samples that could have helped us screen our blood supply that they weren't sharing because they didn't have political permission to do it. So, diplomats clearly intervene to try to get the political framework under which scientists can cooperate more freely. That was certainly the case in the early days of COVID-19 when Chinese scientists were not cooperating with others because they didn't have political permission or space to do so"* (CORE 1).

Global Health Diplomacy Training

While reflecting on specific training for Global Health Diplomacy, a few Core

GHD actors shared specific competencies they believed GHD actors would benefit from

being trained in. The table below presents specific training domains, which include the

ability to understand International Regulations and Governance frameworks, pandemic

preparedness and response, knowing how to negotiate and navigate diplomatic

interactions, as well as leveraging case studies, simulation exercises, mentorship, and

peer-learning to create avenues for practicing and honing these skills:

Table 11

Core GHD Actors' Expression of Global Health Diplomacy Training Domains

Training Domain	CORE GHD Actor Excerpt
International Regulations/ Regulatory Processes and Governance Frameworks	*"The idea is not going to be to give people Nursing 101, or something like that, right? But you still can do 'understanding the basics of the regulatory process for a new investigative drug' and some of those regulatory things that would be very useful. And modules on understanding data flow in a system. It's good to see that the academic community is addressing it and trying to look at how we put this together. It's all part of being better prepared next time. Having the people well trained for it next time, and there will be a next time. [Knowing] what we have in terms of the governance framework as a global community,*

	because it's not important until it is, and then, once it is, it's really, really important, and most people don't know" (CORE 7).
Diplomacy/Diplomatic Interactions	*"The State Department trains their people in the Foreign Service or the Department of Defense. So, as number one, I say, being technically savvy, being a subject matter expert. I wouldn't get a person out of whatever career and make them a Global Health Diplomat, but someone from the health sciences of some kind, language skills are super important, and diplomatic skills and protocol learning are super important. When you go through the State Department, they train you on protocol matters. You know, from how to eat, if you're sitting with senior dignitaries to how to be in a receiving line to understand if you happen to run into them on a bus or an elevator to understand how you address people respectfully. We even learn how to kiss socially when you go to other countries on the cheeks, and we laugh about that. I see people like, 'Oh, my God, I don't want to kiss anybody,' That's the way you're gonna greet people in that country"* (CORE 4).
Pandemic Preparedness / Emergency Response	*"I'm glad you are thinking of a training curriculum because otherwise, you'd have experts around the world with no idea what a global context is; they have no idea what it is to be a diplomat. The type of issues that you're gonna be dealing with in an emergency: strengthening global health security by developing capacities to deploy medical countermeasures internationally gives you a good idea of the things that you need to train people on, so it's very important that we have a new generation that is trained in all the things; liability protections, liability issues, and regulatory issues, logistical issues, that you understand the type of things on the paperwork that you're gonna need to do with a deployment. I think those are gonna give you a good idea of the competencies and specific training"* (CORE 4).
Case Studies and Real-world Simulation Exercises	*"Case studies, role plays, and so on are very important. So, the sense of being familiar with the subject matter and past instances, and where we've been able to successfully combat outbreaks, and where we've made some mistakes, to me, is the best kind of training that you need to be familiar with the worlds of public health and of diplomacy"* (CORE 1). *"I think of the way business school operates where they look at case studies, and I think case studies, particularly when you're looking at things that didn't work well, can be really important. This is very relevant to the context of the negotiations going on in Geneva, where I think a lot of what is being negotiated doesn't account for the real-world complexity. I'm concerned that they're taking some approaches that have worked, some very elegant solutions that have worked well in the influenza world, and they're trying to generalize them, and I'm not convinced that they are actually generalizable, and so I think, being able to take that skeptical eye and say, why won't this work? I think it's a really tough thing"* (CORE 3).

Bilateral and Multilateral Negotiations	*"Some training and rules of order in how to go through multilateral negotiation processes, which is its own bizarre kind of culture that's probably useful, as well as learning how negotiations happen. And learning how to engage in a bilateral and multilateral context"* (CORE 6).
Mentorship and Peer-Learning	*"It's my view that they [competencies] can be picked up through other people's experience. However, not every diplomat has to go through the learning process by himself or herself. There's a there's a body of knowledge in the sense of 'Which these buckets of experiences do this fall?' That's why I was thinking that AIDS really was not a fast-breaking outbreak. This was something we've developed for many years, and by the time it became a priority agenda in Africa, we knew a lot about the virus, and, in fact, by the time PEPFAR started, we had the countermeasure"* (CORE 1).

Understanding Global Health Diplomacy in Practice

While reflecting on the real-world practice of GHD, some Core GHD participants explained the non-linear path that led to some GHD actors becoming present-day Global Health Diplomats:

> *"A lot of Global Health Diplomats became Global Health Diplomats because they were Foreign Service Officers. They were Economic officers in Zambia, Barbados, or Bolivia, and they didn't have any global health people. They were generalists who had to learn really quickly to understand epidemiology, disease, transmission, and statistics. They had to get smart and quick on this stuff. What they had as diplomats was the ability to synthesize information, weed out the critical information and what was unnecessary, and know who to ask questions. And they also had that cultural competency that we talked about because they're diplomats; that's what they're supposed to do. On the other side of it were health people who suddenly had to negotiate treaties, contracts, and stuff, so they needed to quickly understand how to reduce what they had into something palatable"* (CORE 5).

Sharing a similar perspective, another Core GHD actor discussed efforts the State Department was undertaking to build and strengthen the capacity of diplomats and US embassy staff, albeit whilst also arguing that skills required for GHD were not that different from those of a core [non-health] diplomat:

> *"I'm always a little bit uncomfortable with the question that you started with, and many academics are speaking in these terms, about [GHD] skillset, and*

diplomats also do this. The Foreign Service Institute is looking at courses that can impart skills to diplomats or people who work in embassies that will better equip us to do our jobs, and that's good. But it does seem to me that's saying that there's a global health skill set that's different than the core skills that diplomats need. I think what we need in terms of training or capacity building is how do you apply those skills that diplomats would have in general to health problems or health challenges? And how do we look for opportunities in the health sector to advance national security to advance the US or other governments interests or goals that have been defined by either the diplomatic side or the health side" (CORE 1).

Knowledge of Stakeholders and Multisectoral Engagement

Regarding the knowledge and engagement of multisector stakeholders, one Core GHD actor commented on the importance for GHD actors to identify who their key stakeholders are and how to engage with them through participatory approaches to build relationships that can be leveraged across multiple sectors for successful outcomes:

"Knowing your partners, knowing who needs to be at the table, or how to persuade the priority partners for a particular intervention or a particular crisis response based on your knowledge of the local situation of the crisis of the partners. Again, it's a skill that diplomats should have because you're dealing with a number of issues at any one time. Still, the sense of who the public health partners are might be very different from if it's a question of a military nature, or of an economic nature or trade question. The public health partners are likely to include many more civil society groups, perhaps more cultural and religious leaders. You deal with the media in a different way, and you would deal with policymakers in a different way" (CORE 1).

Negotiation

Reflecting on interactions in multilateral settings, Core GHD actors stated that the art of negotiation is a critical, practiced-based competency for GHD actors. One respondent within this category explained the process of negotiation for consensus-building amongst Member States at WHO headquarters. They explained the need for GHD actors to understand the challenges of getting Member States to come to an agreement:

"In Geneva, we would talk about 'the spirit of Geneva,' whereby negotiations at the World Health Assembly are different from most other negotiations in the diplomatic world because there really is an emphasis on consensus. Most of what we do is non-binding; I think there's a recognition that it's frankly very hard to get countries to agree to be bound on a lot of these measures because they do go deep into their domestic issues and their way of doing things. So, this spirit of Geneva is really about trying to come to a consensus in almost every instance, which can be difficult, and you always have to remember that this is non-binding. That it's really meant to encourage. It's intended to point everyone in the right direction without always requiring that they go there. So, I think having that flexibility of understanding is important" (CORE 6).

Understanding Global Governance Frameworks and Multilateral Organizations

When considering global governance frameworks and the way international organizations operate, Core GHD respondents deemed it important for GHD actors to familiarize themselves with global health guidelines, industry standards, and evidence-informed practices, and the host of key multilateral organizations that exercised their influence in this space:

"Understanding the workings of multilateral institutions, like CEPI, Gavi, and other organizations broadly, how they function, how they're made up. What kind of mandates do they have? Are they normative bodies? Are they regulatory bodies? Do they have any enforcement mechanisms? How do those fit together? It's very useful to understand economic organizations where countries are Member States. An example is SADC (Southern Africa Development Community), which has rules for members that are different from other countries. So then, if you have that, then you've sort of committed certain kinds of things about information sharing, immigration access and free mobility, migration, and those things can have a huge impact when you're dealing with an epidemic. So, that kind of economic underlay to the way that we're organized as a planet is very, very useful: ASEAN, SADC, CARICOM, the European Union, those things make a difference. You have to be conversant in them because they will influence how things work" (CORE 7).

Understanding of US Interagency Protocols

While discussing UN interagency protocols, one Core GHD participant accentuated the need for GHD actors to seek to understand the role and responsibilities of each US federal agency, and these may intertwine with the GHD actors' daily activities.

They also recommended an understanding of the interagency coordination framework to maximize impact, resources, and knowledge dissemination when responding to global health threats:

> *"Something [that's] very important; if you're gonna be representing the United States abroad is to have a deep understanding of the US Interagency coordination protocols. You really need to know who the experts are and how to go through the proper channels. You need to be very versatile in all the processes and protocols for United States policymaking. There are slight changes from administration to administration, but you need to understand those roles and what roles they want to play in your work and your day-to-day job because you're gonna be talking to them a lot"* (CORE 4).

4. Learning Competencies

Learning competencies collectively refer to the processes by which GHD actors acquire knowledge, skills, or abilities through a previous experience that leads to positive change to enhance GHD practice. These included GHD actors' ability to learn on the job as the responsibilities of their roles shift, as well as understanding the role that private entities play in global health, which may sometimes be perceived as altruistic or self-serving:

On-the-job Learning

While discussing learning competencies, Core GHD actors recognized the wide range of topics or activities that may arise for which GHD actors have not been formally trained. Some participants highlighted the need for GHD actors to adopt a learning disposition that allowed them to develop new competencies while practicing GHD:

> *"You just have to sort of learn what you can about the [for example] hardware stuff and the technology and then see what other skills you need to know about the atmosphere you're operating in and the challenges you're going through. And these aren't usually technical issues. They're usually ones that are multisectoral where you have to look at how the systems work, what are the economic, the sociological, the ethical challenges of what you're trying to do, and that's even more true, probably of health interventions than even trade, or economic or political or military ones"* (CORE 1).

Another respondent disclosed some advice they shared with their team members on how to deal with unplanned questions or impromptu situations during public diplomatic interactions:

> *"There's a couple of things that I tell my staff: you cannot die of embarrassment, meaning, if you are put on the spot to answer something, you will be fine. The agenda is final when the meeting is over, meaning you may go into a meeting thinking it's gonna go one way; if it goes off, that's fine. Oh, and never try to save the government time or money; you'll lose both* (CORE 5).

Understanding the Role of the Private Sector

Reflecting on the role of the private sector, one Core GHD actor emphasized the role of the private sector as a vital global health actor and provider of essential health services that were critical to the pandemic response. They especially noted the private sector's contribution to the production or development of diagnostics, therapeutics, and other medical supplies that supported the pandemic response. They further added that GHD actors needed to understand the drivers and motivations of the private sector and treat them as they would other key stakeholders with whom they would be negotiating:

> *"All of the medical countermeasures come from the private sector. They're developed by the private sector; they're manufactured by the private sector, and a lot of the supply chain is through the private sector. And I think a lot of people in the public health world, in general, often find the private sector a little bit distasteful. In the US, the one thing that really worked well was Operation Warp Speed because the [Trump] Administration was willing to bring in people who had a private sector outlook on things. When you compare the US approach to the European approach, I remember reading a really nice quote that the US treated the private sector like partners, and Europe treated the private sector like customers. And the result was that we got the vaccines produced at scale and into arms much more quickly than Europe did, so I think understanding the business side of this is really important"* (CORE 3).

5. Communication Competencies

Communication competencies collectively refer to GHD actors' use of various communication formats, such as written and verbal communication, public speaking, elevator pitches, and crisis/risk communication, in GHD practice. Communication was a salient theme for Core GHD Actors, with more than two-thirds of this group insisting on the importance for GHD actors to master a variety of communication formats, as well as the ability to synthesize information so their intended audience can easily understand it:

> *"Writing skills are important, as are speaking and communication skills. You have to use language carefully. You have to know what you know. You have to be able to express uncertainty and deal with risk appropriately, and you have to be able to express that in a way that communicates your message to the public that both reassures but leaves room for change and doubt. So, communication skills, I would say, are at the top"* (CORE 1).

The same respondent further explained how they utilized different approaches to communication in different health emergency scenarios, noting the importance of adapting one's messaging to the specific audience and context:

> *"You certainly need public health expertise; you have to identify exactly what messages you're trying to give to foreign partners. On the other hand, the actual politics of each situation is quite different, and the solutions are different. [For example] in Brazil, it [Zika] was a question of really sitting down with the Minister of Health and just reaching an agreement on a document, which you could do in a day. In Sierra Leone [for Ebola], it took a month of somebody camping out on the steps of the President to say, look, you've got a problem. And I know you don't think you do, but you do. And how are we going to get this message across to you?"* (CORE 1).

Sharing a similar opinion, one Core GHD actor also highlighted the importance of being persuasive, especially when trying to motivate one's counterparts and convince them of mutually beneficial outcomes that may originate from their decisions:

> *"You often don't get very much time with decision-makers when you're in these kinds of things. The decision-makers you talk to often will not have technical expertise, and you need to be able to say the single most important thing. [For instance] we need to convince the government we're working with that they need to share samples of the strain that they found of this virus, here's why they need to do that. And you need to be able to put that into terms that a politician or an ambassador can understand. If I'm going to try to talk to a Minister of Health in another country about this, what is going to motivate him? What is he thinking about? And being sensitive to those motivations. How am I thinking about how*

we're going to allay the concerns that he has? Because these issues are complicated" (CORE 7).

Expounding upon their previous statement, the Core GHD actor went further to explain why acquiring samples was vital for developing vaccines. They also recognized that despite sharing samples, the vaccines or countermeasures developed were sometimes out of the reach of the countries from which these samples were obtained:

> *"We can't make effective vaccines for emerging viruses if we don't have samples of them. However, many countries have very real issues with things that have occurred in the past, and still, unfortunately, occur where they share samples, and then in an industrialized country, the vaccine is purchased, and then they can't afford to give it to their people"* (CORE 7).

Another Core GHD actor highlighted the importance for GHD actors to learn public speaking as they may be called up to fulfill the requirements of a public speaking engagement at short notice about a range of health and non-health topics:

> *"There are many instances where the [US] Ambassador is invited to health events, and obviously, his/her agenda is super busy, and then you go [to represent them], and you need to behave correctly. It's very important to learn public speaking; you are going to be invited by the host country to give a lot of opening remarks at a lot of conferences where you don't know the topic or you are not an expert on that topic. I'm an expert in health security, a scientist before that, but I will go to talk about mental health, drugs, suicide, water, safety, and security. So, you have to be ready to be and able to be a good communicator in general, and then understand the communication style in the country, and it's not just managing the language"* (CORE 4).

For one participant within the Core GHD category, until GHD actors became proficient in public speaking, they needed to cultivate the belief in their ability to deliver and keep on building the skill through repeated practices. They also emphasized the importance of GHD actors being concise and precise whilst delivering their message:

> *"Sometimes, you just have to fake it until you make it and be comfortable with that. Sometimes you're just gonna be thrown into a meeting, either you're representing [the US Ambassador], and you just have to be able to go, 'I can do this,' or you're gonna be briefing somebody, and you need to make sure that that person you're briefing boils down to knowing what's important. We talk about*

BLUF: Bottom Line Upfront, and you need to be able to go, 'okay, here's 5 bullets, and then here's the 6 pages, if you want it" (CORE 5).

Multistakeholder Global Health Diplomacy Actors' Core Competencies

This section presents Multistakeholder GHD actors' expression of core competencies required for Global Health Diplomacy practice. Multistakeholder GHD actors did not share any core competencies related to the critical and analytical thinking theme. However, the findings from the other themes are presented below:

1. **Interpersonal Competencies**

Interpersonal competencies collectively refer to traits and abilities that GHD actors expressed were critical for harmonious interactions with others from diverse cultural backgrounds, facilitating the building and fostering of relationships. Several, Multistakeholder GHD actors highlighted the importance for GHD actors to be aware, considerate, and sensitive to others' cultures, in addition to leading with honesty and transparency and the ability to foster genuine personal connections, which they thought were fundamental personal interactions and building relationships

Cross-cultural Awareness and Cultural Sensitivity

Reflecting on their work during the COVID-19 pandemic response, some respondents within the Multistakeholder actor category shared instances where being culturally competent helped advance their public health goals, by embodying a range of interpersonal traits:

> *"We had individuals who wanted to do things their way, and we had to let them know that we love your passion, but you are part of a larger construct. The big thing is leading them; but in order to lead them effectively where the organization has to go—not just where they want to go, the best way I found is to have a conversation with them, get to know them, and apply all those soft skills that we talk about active-listening, engagement, empathy, humility, servant leadership,*

*adaptability. And then also, when you realize if that person doesn't have the skill
set, how do you get them the skill set in an expeditious manner?" (MSTK 2).*

Another commented on how foreknowledge of behaviors, beliefs, or values of people
from different cultural backgrounds helped guide their interactions to avoid offending
their counterparts or inadvertently committing perceived improprieties:

> *"That [cross-cultural awareness] helps me with my job because when I start
> thinking this person is speaking this particular language, I'm already
> automatically thinking this person may be from this country or that country, so
> what cultures are they part of? How should I approach them? If you know they're
> from a culture that is male-dominant, as a female, I would not want to approach a
> male in a certain way, or I may have to ask permission first from the male in
> order to speak to his wife. So, being culturally sensitive and culturally
> appropriate, I think that kind of comes from languages" (MSTK 4).*

Personable or Soft Skills

One Multistakeholder GHD actor shared some personal traits that created a
foundation for building trusted and genuine diplomatic relationships, albeit recognizing
that these relationships can be underpinned by both positive and negative end results,
which the GHD actor would have to reconcile:

> *"Health diplomacy is successful when it is fueled by honesty, pragmatism,
> realism, and respect. At the heart of diplomacy is a relationship, and you have
> that relationship for both good and bad reasons in the sense that diplomacy is
> about relationships so that you can maintain peace, so that you are able to be a
> negotiator if that's what you need to do at that time. Sometimes, it's actually fun,
> and it is about the exchange of ideas, and it could be in all kinds of sectors, but at
> its core, it is about having a relationship with both your friends and your
> adversaries so that you can solve the problems of the day. And we carve out those
> problems of the day by sectors, regions, or some other parameter" (MSTK 1).*

Transparency

For another Multistakeholder GHD actor, being honest and transparent was the
defining factor for whether non-Whites or 'people of color' enrolled in a COVID-19
study at a time when attempts to recruit study participants were met with heightened
suspicion:

145

"Transparency was paramount. We ended up getting more African Americans into the [COVID research] protocols because [initially] we had issues getting people of color into our protocols. When I was called upon to recruit more persons of color, I was very honest with them. One of the things that I stressed was: 'This is why we need you; we don't have your representation, and I understand why you may be apprehensive about doing this, but here's the reason why we need you in the study, and this is what we're trying to do.' Whenever I used that approach, people were like, where do I sign up? (MSTK 2).

Leadership

Reflecting on competent leadership, one Multistakeholder GHD actor shared leadership tenets they thought were vital for GHD actors while leading teams, particularly in crisis or emergencies. They reiterated the need for leaders to understand how to best motivate their teams by seeking to understand what drives them or what they care about, explaining that these attributes went beyond having the required technical skills:

"Public health is everything that we do, but having an understanding of leadership is critical. And that is not only speaking to people or having the humility and empathy to understand what folks are going through. But in order for you to lead them, you have to figure out what it is that they want to do, and a lot of these individuals were giving of themselves, and all they really wanted to do was to apply their skill sets to help others in need. You can tap into that energy, maneuver their skill sets, and combine them with the overall team concept to further the mission. You can have the technical skills, but having the ability to speak to individuals and persuade them to do what you need them to do is only possible by building a rapport. I can't stress that enough. We often talk about these as soft skills, but they're so hard to do, so they're incredibly important" (MSTK 2).

Partnership development

When sharing about partnership development, one Multistakeholder GHD participant articulated the need for personal credibility and trustworthiness in partnership development, noting that these attributes were key to sustaining partnerships in the long term:

"Being credible, trustworthy, and making sure you gain their [partners'] trust. We've been talking a lot about leadership and partnership, but we know that takes time. All that stuff is not something that can be rushed, so we can't wait till the next pandemic to work on this. If there is another pandemic, we're ready to be credible: a credible face, and a credible voice, and a credible source that other countries, if necessary, can look to, and we can foster diplomacy between different countries. So, I think that's a really critical part: gaining the trust of the people you work with and gaining the trust of your partners is going to be very, very important. I think sustainability is also a critical component because you can make a decision, or you could be diplomatic about something with one individual or whatever partners are at the table, but that doesn't mean it's going to continue" (MSTK 4)

2. Technical Competencies

Technical competencies collectively refer to specialized expertise that GHD actors can leverage while practicing Global Health Diplomacy. This section presents specialized technical expertise that Multistakeholder GHD actors expressed as being important for Global Health Diplomacy practice in a post-COVID era.

The table below captures Multistakeholder GHD actors' expressions of technical competencies required for practicing Global Health Diplomacy. Respondents highlighted emergency preparedness and response, monitoring and evaluating projects, generating after-project reports, and the ability to utilize and manage data systems. Multistakeholder GHD actors also emphasized the importance of GHD actors having global or public expertise.

Table 12

Multistakeholder GHD actors' expression of required technical competencies for GHD practice

Technical Area	GHD Actor Excerpt
Project Reporting, Monitoring, and Evaluation	*"Reporting and M&E are really important. I think there's a lot of preparation that needs to go into changing how we work as an organization globally, how we preposition funds, how we make financing available to countries earlier, and how we also evaluate our work"* (MSTK 3).

	"Also, being able to use that data after the pandemic or the outbreak has passed to figure out how you can do things better and how you can improve. Sometimes, those recommendations are just theories, and they might not actually work and might take more LOE [level of effort] to implement than you might have" (MSTK 3).
Data Systems and Management	*"It's all about the data systems. Sometimes, the data systems in particular countries are not particularly strong or do not have the infrastructure that would work for us to collect the data we need. So, during COVID, there were a lot of investments in new data systems and data systems that were made interoperable between existing data systems. But again, it's really hard. A lot of money is thrown into data, so I think we can really do a better job there"* (MSTK 3).
Expertise in Scientific, Clinical or Technical Intricate Area	*Training in pathogens and in epidemiology and laboratory, and that sort of thing. To be a Global Health Diplomat, it's important that you have a content area, whether it's HIV, or it's TB, or it's malaria, or it's laboratories, or it's outbreak investigations, where you bring to the table a certain skill set that is desirable. And through that relationship, you create trust, and that trust is really the diplomacy"* (MSTK 7).
Emergency Preparedness and Response	*"Whatever technical skills are needed to respond to that particular outbreak. If you're looking at Global Health Diplomacy, maybe it's even laboratory knowledge becoming really important. Knowing how things are going to be tested and when they're going to be tested. How do we strengthen the last-mile laboratory systems in certain countries?"* (MSTK 3)
Global Health / Public Health	*"I would say number one. First and foremost, as we have been taught, public health is everywhere. Public health is everything that we do"* (MSTK 2) *" I would argue that you can't be a global health diplomat without some competency in global health. I think that the whole point of relationships that include an element of trust is that you can talk to me about medical countermeasures in the health space, and I would have the confidence that what you're arguing for is coming out of some knowledge base that you have "* (MSTK 1).

3. Practical or Practice-Based Competencies

This section presents Multistakeholder GHD actors' expression of practical competencies applied in real-world GHD settings or Global Health Diplomacy competencies in action. Respondents emphasized the need for real-world experience in the field of GHD and an appraisal of the contexts in which actors will be engaging with others. They also proposed specific training areas they felt were critical for GHD actors.

Contextual and Situational Awareness

While discussing the importance of contextual and situational awareness, one Multistakeholder GHD study participant accentuated the need for GHD actors to maintain a heightened awareness of the countries and contexts in which they found themselves. The respondent further noted the power imbalance that consciously or unconsciously skews negotiations between GHD actors who held the purse strings and their counterparts on the receiving end of foreign assistance:

> *"It is very hard for people to respect [others] when they have a checkbook because they think that that's actually what matters. I encourage partners when we're talking, I say, feel free to say no to us, feel free to actually say, 'That doesn't work for me, this is where I wanna go,' because many times, the partner countries who are engaged in an exercise with us have numerous people who have something they want and when you are without resources, you feel you don't have the kind of agency. I tell people, you actually have every bit of agency; this is your country. When our team starts talking in a meeting with the [host] government and talking about 'our sites,' I'm like, okay, that is someone who does not have situational awareness because, at that point, you stopped having a relationship. The people [from the host government] are not actually talking to you right now because they're like, 'What the heck is that?' They're not saying it, but it's in there"* (MSTK 1).

The same Multistakeholder GHD actor invited GHD actors to frequently assess their biases and assumptions about the people they worked with, as well as whether their expertise was still useful within a given setting:

> *"Being very clear in your mind that when you are an outsider coming to work in another person's country, you have to identify the problem, and you have to have a path to solving it. It can't be that you view your partner as having endless problems, and you always being in a relationship where you're the fixer. So, for me, this whole concept in global health around technical assistance is a double-edged sword in some ways that could actually get misconstrued where you like that [dependency] framework, but the person in receipt of it is probably capable of doing that [technical aspect]"* (MSTK 1).

Global Health Diplomacy Training

Reflecting on the need for GHD training, some Multistakeholder GHD actors shared specific training competencies they felt would be useful for Global Health Diplomacy actors. In the table below, respondents' expressions of competency training domains reflect the GHD actors' proficiency in emergency preparedness and response, global health security, public health, health policy, and interpersonal interactions. The Multistakeholder GHD actors also mentioned the need for cross-cultural exchanges and mentorship for GHD actors in a post-COVID era.

Table 13

Multistakeholder GHD Actors Expression of Required Competency Training Domains

Training Domain	GHD Actor Excerpt
Emergency Preparedness and Response	*"We've been working on some tabletop exercises where we have a scenario and play out the scenario to test our emergency response capabilities as a division or organization. It's become really important to have those exercises because we learned so much from the COVID-19 pandemic. We want to be able to exercise those skills and knowledge across the organization to understand where gaps might be and where challenges or conflicts might come into play in advance of actually responding to an emergency in the health area"* (MSTK 3). *" Preparedness involves many different stakeholders, is quite complex, and involves funding. So, it's important to consider that it's not going to be a one-size-fits-all when we offer suggestions on how to strategize or prepare for an outbreak"* (MSTK 3).
Global Health Security	*"We're also looking at spreading knowledge around global health security through training, getting everyone up to speed, and having a general level of knowledge"* (MSTK 3).
Public Health and Health Policy	*" I think if you had a set of people in front of you to train, you want them to be really good public health scientists and very flexible"* (MSTK 3). *"And so being effective in those diplomatic aspects of health policy and practice"* (MSTK 5).
Mentoring and Cross-Cultural Exchanges	*"Other types of training that might be more beneficial [would be] cross-collaboration learning across different missions, learning across different positions in an organization. Mentoring and exchanges with missions where someone would*

	come and be at IHQ for three months and then go back to the field, so, we learn from them, and they learn from us, and they transfer skills in that way" (MSTK 3).
Interpersonal Training	*"All the leadership and team-building training: how to work in a team and collaborate, what it means to lead, and what it means to be a partner? All those things, I think, are some of those core competencies"* (MSTK 3).

Global Health Diplomacy Practice or Practical Experience

While reflecting on the practice of GHD in real-world settings, one

Multistakeholder GHD actor commented on the transition of Foreign Service Officers to

become Global Health Diplomats. They divulged that most Foreign Service Officers

stationed at US Embassies abroad often did not have a public health or scientific

background, although they had other non-health related expertise from their dedicated

foreign service career tracks:

> *"It's an interesting thing because, in the Embassy world, many people who get certain jobs may not always have a background in that area. So, the Science and Environmental officer, or whatever that title is, has foreign service training, but they may not be a biologist or a scientist or whatever, and certainly, they're really unlikely to have public health training; I'd say that's probably very unusual. And so when they go meet, say, a Minister of Health, they go into this meeting because they have a high-level US government position and a certain authority because of that, but not because of their content knowledge. They have it because of their position in a different institution, like the CDC or other institutions in these same countries, from a technical perspective. They have training in pathogens, epidemiology, laboratory, and that sort of thing. So, when they meet the Ministry of Health, they meet that person or those people through a technical path, and that path creates diplomacy"* (MSTK 7).

Another Multistakeholder GHD actor shared their experience about the strategic

influence that GHD actors have, which they said was just as important as the role the

military might play when engaging with foreign governments:

> *"When Secretary Clinton was the Secretary of State, she would pull us into that space she called her soft power. We didn't have weapons, we didn't have military*

hardware, but it was equally important what was possible through our channels"
(MSTK 1).

The same respondent further discussed the strengths of Global Health Diplomacy as

critical to US foreign policy, multisectoral cooperation and collaboration, articulating

how health for diplomacy can be employed for building peace and a window into other

cultures:

> *"It's the coolest thing because we work with a lot of ambassadors, our
> ambassadors, other diplomats in the department, and health colleagues, and
> when we get asked to help problem-solve, you realize that you have this
> unbelievable asset. Health diplomacy is actually a very critical tool in the US
> Toolbox of helping to create world peace. It's a powerful tool of our foreign
> policy, and I think the reason why people feel good about it is because you're
> helping people. This area often bridges gaps, and it helps inform each other about
> the similarities of our cultures. Those similarities connect us, that this is about
> improving the lives of people"* (MSTK 1).

Weighing in on the importance of building and fostering relationships, another

Multistakeholder GHD actor commented on how trusted relationships underpin Global

Health Diplomacy:

> *"When you talk about health, it's really important that there's a trusted
> relationship, and that trusted relationship comes from having worked together,
> and you know something, and then you contribute that something. So, to me,
> there's no such thing exactly as a Global Health Diplomat separate from a global
> health partner with whom you have a relationship"* (MSTK 7).

For another Multistakeholder GHD actor, these relationships are primarily driven by the

GHD actors' general attitude and disposition, both in how they viewed and presented

their issues and how they approached problems presented to them. They argued that

while GHD might be a means for solving issues that transcend the health sector, Global

Health Diplomats need to continuously reassess their relevance to these relationships and

the nature of their engagement within these contexts.

*"Every health diplomat has to believe that the problems you're being confronted
with will have a solution. Or that the people who are on the other side of you,
participating, also want to be independent of your help if that's how it's even
perceived, and that that you have to keep evolving, and you have to keep asking
questions, including, should I still be here participating in this manner? I think
the practice of health diplomacy has to be embedded in solving the problems in
health or all of the health of human beings and bringing that kind of specialized
experience is incredibly helpful. It is a vehicle through which we solve problems
broader than the health sector"* (MSTK 1).

Knowledge of Stakeholders & Stakeholder Engagement

The knowledge and engagement of GHD actors was a salient sub-theme for

Multistakeholder GHD actors. Participants within this group reflected on various aspects

of diplomatic stakeholder interactions, including knowing who the key national and

multinational stakeholders are and the influence they wield in the health sector and across

other sectors. One Multistakeholder GHD actor said:

*"And I think it's a core competency for Global Health Diplomacy, which requires
a lot of research on your end, not just research the situation and take analyses or
assessments of the situation, but also, if I can use the word research individuals
that you are engaging with in a specific way: knowing who you are and who's at
the table"* (MSTK 6).

Sharing a similar perspective, another Multistakeholder GHD actor added the need for

GHD actors' introspection on how and what they might be able to contribute to ongoing

deliberations or negotiations:

*"It's something that's being thought of now and redefined, and responsibilities are
being negotiated in some ways. So, it's really important to understand what
stakeholders are involved and their specific value adds to the conversation. So,
what position do I have in my organization? What does my organization add?
What do we do really well? And then what do our other organizations within the
US Government and beyond do really well that we can rely on?* (MSTK 3).

The same respondent also commented on the noticeable expansion within the US GHD

stakeholder pool. They mentioned that more actors from US federal agencies wanted to actively participate in these multisectoral engagements around health, especially in the

wake of the recent pandemic:

> *"I think it involves more stakeholders; at this point, more departments within the US government want to become engaged in the conversation. We're trying to figure out where everyone fits and then trying to grow each side's capability and strength in those areas"* (MSTK 3).

3. **Learning Competencies**

This section presents Multistakeholder GHD actors' expressions of the process

through which GHD actors acquire knowledge, information, or skills through previous

experience that leads to positive change to build competence and enhance practice, such

as learning on the job. Multistakeholder GHD actors highlighted the need for continuous

learning to build skill and competence in other technical areas and for GHD actors to be

fast learners:

On-the-job Learning

More than half of the Multistakeholder GHD actors emphasized the importance of

continuous learning for GHD actors, especially in technical areas relevant to their roles

that they may not be conversant in:

> *"The general diplomat or a trade diplomat, or a human rights diplomat may not know that technical aspect [related to global health], but they will learn. Again, we're talking about intelligent people who are very smart. At the end of the day, it's a select group of people who will learn, but why wait for that learning process while they can actually know some of these basic things or be aware of them?"* (MSTK 6).

Another Multistakeholder GHD actor added that prior to the COVID-10 pandemic, no

one was an expert on the novel coronavirus and thus had to learn about it, to better

understand how best to contain or mitigate its spread:

> *"Being fluent in specific health policies and factors. No one was an expert on SARS-CoV-2 before 2020, and you don't really need to be a population ecologist or molecular biologist to be effective in that context. So, I think people who have*

those kinds of ongoing learning skills and are able to seek out, learn, and use good information sources had an advantage" (MSTK 5).

One Multistakeholder GHD actor asserted that the onus was on GHD actors to identify their weaknesses and take the necessary actions to fill those. Another participant within this group called for GHD actors' reflection and objectivity during the learning process by leveraging lessons from prior infectious disease outbreaks:

> *"Learning, being reflective, and analyzing what worked well, what could we have done better? And then preparing for the future, not waiting until the next pandemic. What we're trying to do better now is to learn from the COVID pandemic, what we did from our responses to Marburg and Ebola; learning from those responses to inform future responses, to strengthen how we do things"* (MSTK 3).

4. **Communication Competencies:**

Communication competencies collectively refer to GHD actors' use of various communication formats, such as written and verbal communication, public speaking, elevator pitches, and crisis/risk communication, in GHD practice. A few Multistakeholder GHD actors expressed the need for GHD actors to be effective communicators, reiterating that this competency was particularly useful for generating a rapport between partners, building trust, and clarifying uncertainty:

> *"Knowing how to communicate concisely, accurately, using the best information you have in a timely manner can be really hard when you're dealing with limited information. When you're dealing with stakeholders who might not be sharing information or information that's changing minute to minute or hour to hour. So, I think communication is really important, both internally within an organization and externally"* (MSTK 3).

Another respondent within this group stated that while they didn't think everyone needed to be a trained communicator, GHD actors needed to know how to interact with other people, especially across cultures:

> *"Sometimes, we get people who go to countries who are very skilled technically, but they don't know how to have a relationship with the people that they have*

*gone to help, and then it looks like you've come to execute a project.
Communication is super, super important, and just simple things, such as 'maybe
I'm gonna ask some questions first, rather than tell people what it is they need or
want,' which I got to experience firsthand"* (MSTK 1).

Another Multistakeholder GHD actor added: *"I feel diplomacy should require that you
have some sort of [foreign] language background or linguistic background* (MSTK 4).

Informal Global Health Diplomacy Actors' Core Competencies

This section presents Informal GHD actors' expression of core competencies
required for Global Health Diplomacy practice. The Informal GHD actors did not share
any core competencies as pertains to the Technical, Critical and Analytical Thinking, and
Learning Competencies themes, most likely because they had already discussed sub-
themes whilst answering the previous research questions. However, the findings for the
other three themes have been presented below.

1. **Interpersonal Competencies**

Interpersonal competencies collectively refer to traits and abilities that GHD
actors expressed were critical for harmonious interactions with others from diverse
cultural backgrounds to facilitate the building and fostering of relationships. While
discussing this theme, Informal GHD actors underscored the importance of leadership
and transparency as critical to Global Health Diplomacy.

Leadership

Half of the respondents in this category mentioned leadership as a core
competency for GHD actors in combination with other people skills such as
trustworthiness, honesty, credibility, and transparency:

> *"I mentioned servant leadership [very specifically]. You need to have a strong
> work ethic, somebody who understands that this job [in emergency responses]is
> not a 9-to-5, and it's not going to be successful if you are just bound to a 9-to-5.*

156

> *Also, self-confidence: You have to feel confident that you are creating a project and that it can work and be able to convey that to somebody else"* (INFML 7).

Another Informal GHD actor stated the need for calmness, composure, sincerity, and active listening as valuable interpersonal attributes for GHD actors:

> *"A health diplomat needs to be a good listener. They need to be able to be calm, composed, comprehensive, and come out as sincere in trying to engage with their counterparts at the country level when they're engaging in Global Health Diplomacy or even if they are actually engaging at a global level with another organization"* (INFML 6).

Transparency

While reflecting on relevant personality traits, another participant asserted the need for transparency and honesty for GHD actors, adding that they also need to be qualified and able to communicate their knowledge and expertise adequately:

> *"You have to be trustworthy, be honest and transparent. You have to have legitimacy; you have to have the qualifications, and you have to be able to communicate"* (INFML 3)

2. **Practical or Practice-Based Competencies**

This section presents Informal GHD actors' expression of core competencies required for GHD practice in real-world settings or Global Health Diplomacy competencies in action. Informal GHD actors emphasized the need for training across several domains, which include but are not limited to the One Health approach, and understanding the workings of political, governmental, and non-governmental systems, and the contexts in which they were intervening. They also highlighted the knowledge and engagement of stakeholders and the importance of practical experience in Global Health Diplomacy.

Global Health Diplomacy Training

Informal GHD actors also divulged specific training domains that they felt GHD actors needed to build competence in a post-COVID era. The table below presents Informal GHD actors' expressions of specific domains they would like to see GHD actors trained in to make them better practitioners. This group of actors underscores the need for an understanding of how political systems, governments, and non-governmental organizations' function, as well as the ability to understand individual country contexts and the psychological underpinnings of Global Health Diplomacy. Informal GHD actors also emphasized the need for the GHD and public health workforce to be trained in public health and Essential Public Health functions. They further noted that this new era calls for more interdisciplinary training and a revision of medical schools and public health schools' curricula to include the One Health approach and other recent scientific discoveries or contributions:

Table 14

Informal GHD Actors' Expression of GHD Training Domains Required for GHD Practice

Training Domain	GHD Actor Excerpt
Functioning of Political Systems	*"I think if somebody's to walk into a Global Health Diplomacy Masters or Ph.D. Programs at Georgetown should include the political systems, how political systems work, how political actors think, and what they do. How do they react? How do they all fit together within countries, but also between countries? So, you're not gonna know everything, but you can create those little bits of foundation within the system so that a person is aware of financing, communications, culture, politics, political systems, how political actors move or don't move, why they react and don't react"* (INFML 5).
Governmental and Non-Governmental Organizations	*"I think obviously an understanding of the iNGO [International NGO] world is important. But also understanding the different actors that are not only governmental but also the private sector, the iNGO, and the NGO sector"* (INFML 5). *"I think people really need to understand what NGO roles are. If you work for a government agency, it's a heavy lift, and you don't*

	have to depend just on yourself. So, having knowledge of doing a stakeholder analysis is really important as well" (INFML 1)
Communication	*"Having a good understanding of communications in the 2020s. Where we are dealing with information within the fractured network of communication where so many different platforms exist. How do you function in that environment where it's so difficult to get your message across? So, I think understanding how to communicate, and that's not a linear issue"* (INFML 5).
Industrial Psychology	*"Understanding how publics are moved or not moved Global Health Diplomats have too little industrial psychology. They have to understand how individuals and systems think, how they move, how they act, and how they relate. So, a bit of industrial psychology in there would be useful and then optional"* (INFML 5).
Project Management	*"Project management skills training is extremely important"* (INFML 5).
Public Health/ Global Health/ Health Economics	*"Public health is going to be critically important, and an understanding of the economics of how international financial systems move or don't move, and how countries act or do not react in terms of their financial systems is important because that's what's going to pay the bills. And that's what's going to be a prime motivator or obstacle to a Global Health Diplomat's ability to move things forward"* (INFML 5). *"It is always good for people who actually engage in health diplomacy to have some sort of a health background because not all of them do. Or an economic background as a health economist; those things are all important. Obviously, everybody's not gonna be a public health expert, although, in some countries, they actually do have Health Attachés, and so I think that it's important to see what they are trained in and how they can be helpful in this context"* (INFML 6).
Interdisciplinary Education	*"I hope Georgetown sees the magic that it has within its hallowed halls to know that they are poised in a remarkable place to be able to bring together the Walsh schools, you know, as I mentioned before, School of Diplomacy, Global Health, Business, Public Administration into an integrated discipline of Global Health Diplomacy that can actually show many in the rest of the world how to train the individuals for today and tomorrow, who will need to acquire those skills to have the impact to address the complex challenges that we are faced with. Without those skills, then we're not going to be able to translate the technical and scientific discoveries that we have to improve the well-being of people"* (INFML 5).
Country Capacities and Context	*"Understanding the context of the country, the health capacity in the country, the public health capacity, their ability to diagnose and respond, the workforce capacity in the country, and the beliefs of the policymakers about their own country are important and should be included as part of the training"* (INFML 6).

Essential Public Health Functions	*"From my experience of being in global health, individuals, especially those from a US-based training on global health, when you mention Essential Public Health functions, it completely goes over their heads. They have no concept of what those 12 functions could possibly even be. So, even just getting a baseline would be good for all global health and public health practitioners to have"* (INFML 4).
Integration of Essential Public Health Functions into Public Health Training	*"How do you even apply the Essential Public Health Functions into education and training? How do you even know who the practitioners are that should be doing these functions? And then it really is a more living cycle of constantly reviewing and updating and making sure that we're the most relevant in all of these spheres throughout the future of public health. Because it changes, and it is going to need to change based on the context of the world and where the state of the world is"* (INFML 4).
Public Health Workforce Training and Accreditation	*"Anything that builds the capacity of the public health workforce and prepares them more for the future. For prospective public health practitioners, we have time now to update training institutes' competencies and curriculums to prepare them for what's to come. And for the current practitioners, we have time to build continuing education institutes and training programs to better prepare them. Our field really needs to have a learning mindset, and we're constantly needing to update our skill set and our knowledge. By creating this professionalization pathway, we're hoping that will allow more institutions to integrate the recommendations for the updated Essential Public Health functions and therefore, produce more competent and prepared professionals to join the global health workforce (INFML 4)*
One Health and Recent Scientific Breakthroughs	*"I think schools of public health need to update their curricula to meet these demands for the twenty-first century, and they're very resistant. There's a lot more interest in One Health now than there was ten years ago. Certainly, young people are very interested in it, but that still doesn't change the curriculum to meet the needs of 21st-century public health. I would argue that the medical school curriculum needs to be updated to incorporate some of the scientific breakthroughs of the twenty-first century as well"* (INFML 3).

Knowledge of Stakeholders & Stakeholder Engagement

Informal GHD actors stated that knowing and engaging with other GHD stakeholders within host countries can facilitate gathering critical information that allows GHD actors to better understand whom they were interacting with and what their counterparts' equities were. They added that this mastery ultimately helps the GHD actors understand the political landscape in which they found themselves and hopefully see

things from the perspective of the policy or decision maker:

> *"They need to know who are the prime actors at the country level that they need to engage with, or the policymakers, and also understand and try to gather information on what is the party line of those major actors or policymakers from their own country perspective so that we understand them better before you engage with them in a diplomatic way, to make positive changes to a global health emergency or a response within their own country"* (INFML 6).

Global Health Diplomacy Practice or Practical Experience

When discussing the relevance of practical GHD experience, one Informal GHD

actor emphasized the need for GHD actors to understand and differentiate between

diplomatic objectives for health outcomes and leveraging health outcomes for diplomacy

before entering negotiations. They stressed the importance of understanding negotiating

parties' motivations and aspirations before engaging in negotiations:

> *"And people need to understand that you have diplomacy for health and then health for diplomacy. They really need to understand the difference between the two because sometimes people use health as the way to get other measures taken care of, and you may or may not have time for that, but you need to really understand it so that you don't get frustrated during the process"* (INFML 1).

However, another participant insisted that GHD actors' core competencies would be

defined by US foreign policy priorities, which made it challenging for them to know in

advance what the required core competencies are:

> *"And then again, you can't plan for those competencies if the White House is not interested at all in climate change. That goes to the problems that we have with domestic politics: We can't agree about what we need or want to do"* (INFML 2).

3. **Communication Competencies**

Communication competencies collectively refer to GHD actors' use of various

communication formats, such as written and verbal communication, public speaking,

elevator pitches, and crisis/risk communication, in GHD practice. Half of the Informal

GHD actors underscored the importance of GHD actors being competent in various communication formats. They asserted that communication was the vehicle through which negotiations, leadership, and diplomacy occurred:

> *"Communication is certainly critical; I can't stress enough how important that is. If you're gonna be a diplomat, you certainly have to be skilled in negotiation; you have to be a skilled speaker. Communication is key. You have to be a good communicator, whether through speaking, writing, or meetings. Diplomacy and negotiation are very important. It's all communication leadership"* (INFML 3).

Meanwhile, one Informal GHD actor commented on the use of singing as a form of communication sometimes used by Community Health Volunteers. Another Informal GHD actor accentuated risk communication as a critical ability of GHD actors, considering the fear, mistrust, and uncertainty that characterize global health emergencies:

> *"How they [GHD actors] actually learn to communicate is important because risk communication is also a skill set in itself; you know what you know, you don't know what you don't know, and how to communicate that without being an alarmist. But at the same point in time, be transparent and be forthcoming. Try to be honest and sincere, which your body language should also show. Obviously, there's a lot to be said about how you communicate, and the risk communication piece has become really important"* (INFML 6).

Research Question 3: What technical knowledge gaps exist amongst Global Health Diplomacy actors?

The results for identified gaps in GHD technical knowledge are presented sequentially for each GHD actor category, beginning with the Core, Multistakeholder, and Informal categories. Global Health Diplomacy actors' technical knowledge gaps have been distilled into seven (7) main thematic groups (with sub-themes where applicable) and operationalized as follows:

1. **Systemic Gaps** collectively refers to GHD actors' expression of gaps within public health, political, governance, or regulatory systems that resulted in a sub-optimal response to the COVID-19 pandemic.

2. **Interpersonal Knowledge Gaps** collectively refer to knowledge gaps in traits and abilities that GHD actors expressed were critical for harmonious interactions with others from diverse cultural backgrounds, facilitating the building and fostering of relationships.

3. **Technical, Intricate, or Expert Area Knowledge Gaps** collectively refer to knowledge gaps in specialized or intricate areas that GHD actors can leverage while practicing GHD.

4. **Critical and Analytical Thinking Knowledge Gaps** refer to gaps in GHD actors' knowledge of how to synthesize, analyze, and evaluate information in an objective and logical manner to make informed and sound decisions.

5. **Practical or Practice-Based Knowledge Gaps** refer to GHD actors' expression of technical knowledge gaps while practicing Global Health Diplomacy.

6. **Learning Knowledge Gaps** collectively refer to technical knowledge gaps in the processes by which GHD actors acquire knowledge, information, or skills through a previous experience that leads to positive change that enhances practice.

7. **Communication Knowledge Gaps** collectively refer to gaps in GHD actors' knowledge of the use of various communication formats, such as written,

verbal, public speaking, elevator pitches, and crisis/risk communication, in
GHD practice.

Core Global Health Diplomacy Actors' Technical Knowledge Gaps

This section presents Core GHD actors' expression of technical knowledge gaps
in the practical or theoretical understanding of Global Health Diplomacy, presented
according to the aforementioned themes.

1. **Systemic Gaps**

Systemic gaps collectively refer to GHD actors' expression of gaps within public
health, political, governance, or regulatory systems that resulted in a sub-optimal
response to the COVID-19 pandemic. Within this theme, Core GHD actors discussed the
lack of resources and infrastructure in public health and human resource shortages during
the pandemic that negatively affected pandemic response efforts. They also noted the
effects these gaps had on equitable access to essential resources, information, vaccines,
and therapeutics.

Public Health Resources and Infrastructure

While reflecting on the limited public health infrastructure and the lack of
resources to respond to the COVID pandemic, some Core GHD actors spotlighted the
socioeconomic disparities and health inequities that for so long had gone unaddressed
within the US and in other countries:

> *"COVID-19 really exposed how inequitable the US healthcare system really was.
> I mean we're in healthcare, we knew it, we absolutely knew it. But this really
> picked up the rock, so to speak. I think it also taught us that we need to strengthen
> healthcare systems in a way that is equitable. In the World Health Organization,
> if you ask a hundred countries what they want out of their healthcare system, they
> want equitable, accessible, effective, and easy to pay for, regardless of where they
> are on the socioeconomic scale. I think it [the pandemic] has also, unfortunately,
> worn out our healthcare workers. And so, before the next pandemic comes, we*

need to figure out what kind of health workforce we need and how we're going to get it, and this is true for every country" (CORE 5).

One Core GHD actor said the inadequacies and inconsistencies in the pandemic response also resulted from the lack of Foreign Service Officers at US embassies who were adequately equipped to handle the multifaceted demands of a pandemic response:

> *"We have a workforce that's permanently looking at economic elements, political elements, consular affairs, or management affairs in a country, but we don't have permanent public health staff. If there's no CDC, NIH, or USAID health officers, it's the Economic officer that will play that role without any public health training or the medical officer, and medical officers are clinicians. They're designed to attend to the health needs and the status of that country. They're not really trained in public health, nor do they have the mission to go out and represent the US Government's interest in public health to another government; they're internally focused. So, the core function of an embassy, I would posit, needs to include public health, and it doesn't"* (CORE 2).

Human Resource or Staffing Gaps

Regarding the insufficiency of human resource personnel, one Core GHD actor explained how staffing shortages affected the flow of communication and impeded the US diplomatic mission abroad at a time when having their presence in the country was most crucial:

> *"It's not necessarily that we didn't have the knowledge or technical competence in the bilateral mission in the US Embassy in [location redacted]; it's just that we lacked staff. During the period I was there, the CDC just closed their offices; they just didn't fill the US direct-hire medical officers or epidemiologists, and they slowly pulled their budget. Had we had those positions there, I think we would have had this really robust ability to have informal communication with [redacted foreign location] at a time that was super, super important"* (CORE 2).

The same respondent expounded further on how staffing vacancies also contributed to the supply chain challenges, limiting the US' ability to get critical PPE supplies and resources required for the pandemic response:

> *"When COVID happened, they [the US embassy] evacuated a hundred percent of their staff, all the Americans went home. Then the embassy realized that we had*

this critical supply problem; we didn't have enough masks in the United States. We had critical drugs that weren't being produced that we couldn't get from China, and nobody in the embassy knew how to solve this problem. All of the people who had their counterparts in the Chinese Government were here in the United States, and it was just the perfect storm of cutting off our ability to talk, our ability to see, and our ability to hear around critical supply chains. So again, it was not having the people; it wasn't necessarily that they didn't have the competencies" (CORE 2)

The Core GHD actor also explained how the lack of staff in the host country also significantly restricted US GHD actors and embassy personnel's ability to participate in face-to-face engagements, which are integral to building and fostering diplomatic relationships. They explained that these interactions vary by cultural and situational context and require that GHD actors be immersed into the host culture to learn how these societies function:

> *"There's no substitute for in-person relationships. It is absolutely critical that leaders meet and develop a rapport. That's why we build these in-person meetings into these international negotiations: it's just not possible over a webinar to simulate this and have a real connection between humans. And that relationship can make everything go very smoothly over the next year. We can get concessions that we never would have thought possible if the two leaders are able to get along and negotiate themselves. Thorny issues like sample sharing, data sharing, and issues that really needed to get through our two systems, which were not compatible directly. [For instance], the US CDC system is very different than Chinese CDC system. They function differently. They have different processes, it's not intuitive, and without people on the ground to help guide this diplomatic intercourse, it doesn't function. You won't know sitting in Atlanta what's really going on, and vice versa"* (CORE 2).

The same respondent asserted that many of these relationships take years to build and require that strategically assigned GHD actors maintain a sustained presence in-country to cultivate them, thus preserving formal communication channels:

> *"It takes people with the knowledge, skills, and competencies in public health and diplomacy to be in the right place and at the right time. For critical positions, temporary duty going back and forth during collaborations really has significant limits. You have to be resident there for at least 2-6 years. Those were the limiting factors: the actual number of staff strategically placed. When COVID came, our*

*government lacked the ears and the eyes to know what was going on in order to
find those areas of mutual interest that would advance our [US] interests. When
you advance our [US] interest in public health, that's going to advance the
world's interests"* (CORE 2).

The Core GHD actor reaffirmed that the lack of critical staff resulted in a missed

opportunity for bilateral cooperation and collaboration and the inability to understand

some of the reasons behind COVID-19 vaccine hesitancy across these populations:

*"I think we could have collaborated on critical functions of epidemic detection
and response, such as sharing information, sharing biospecimens, understanding
how vaccine efficacy was working in the real world as we vaccinated our
populations, understanding vaccine hesitancy in the two populations of the two
largest economies on the planet, and the two largest vaccine production efforts on
the planet. We could have been a little bit more strategic with this"* (CORE 2).

Limited Research and Publication in GHD Competencies

Reflecting on the role of research in Global Health Diplomacy, one GHD actor

also mentioned that GHD actors' knowledge, skills, and competencies were largely

unexplored due to limited research and scholarship in this area:

*"There's an aspect of research diplomacy, there's not many people that publish
on the competencies around global health diplomacy. It's a nascent field around
the practice of health diplomacy, and I really welcome your analytical work. I
think it's much needed; it's very timely, I think"* (CORE 2).

2. **Interpersonal Knowledge Gaps**

This section presents knowledge gaps in the traits and abilities that Core GHD

actors expressed were critical for harmonious interactions with others from diverse

cultural backgrounds to build and foster relationships, such as working or collaborating

within a team.

Collaboration and Teamwork

Reflecting on the events of the recent pandemic, one Core GHD actor

underscored the need for bilateral and multilateral collaboration among GHD actors for a stronger and more coordinated pandemic response, even as countries strove to pursue their own priorities. This respondent described the benefits of countries sharing viral samples, data, and resources at a time when the virus was spreading rapidly:

> *"Countries went to their own national interests, first and foremost, which we [the US] did as well. From a public health standpoint, it's incumbent upon us to be able to identify areas where it's in our benefit to collaborate, allowing samples, biospecimens to go through borders, allowing data to be exchanged freely, allowing medical supplies in and out, allowing medical teams over borders; all of that became almost impossible, and those were the elements that were just critical during COVID"* (CORE 2).

3. **Technical, Intricate, or Expert Area Knowledge Gaps**

While discussing technical knowledge gaps amongst GHD actors, Core GHD actors expressed several knowledge gaps displayed by a lack of theoretical or practical understanding of intricate or technical areas during GHD practice. In the table below, Core GHD actors highlight the gaps in knowledge of supply chain management and explained how the inability to manage supply chains made it challenging to secure, produce, and distribute essential resources when they were most needed. They also noted that most countries did not have the legal framework for dealing with the liabilities of administering a new drug or vaccine in emergencies, whose effects had not been studied at the individual and population over time. Respondents in this group also emphasized the need for GHD actors to have a clinical or public/global health background, as well as technical expertise in a wide range of technical areas, including knowledge and understanding of global health instruments, regulations, and treaties, foreign policy, and knowledge of how to carry out performance or capacity assessments amongst others.

Table 15

Core GHD Actors' Expression of Technical Knowledge Gaps in GHD Practice

Technical Knowledge Gap	CORE GHD Actor Excerpt
Supply Chain Management	*"Supply chain was what killed us under COVID. Lack of redundancy of supply chain, Lack of understanding of that lack of redundancy, lack of ability to rapidly adapt to that. It takes too long to get new drugs, vaccines, and technologies approved. That's a technical process gap, and we don't have enough ways to manage that."* (CORE 7). *"I don't think we were prepared for some of the supply chain issues. And truly understanding that we have all of these treaties, and they say we're gonna share this, and we're gonna share that. I think we didn't understand contract law, and in the process, we forgot to look at the fine print of the contracts, So I feel like those were some places where we fell down"* (CORE 5).
Clinical, Global Health or Public Health Expertise	*"At the highest level, I cannot insist enough on having health experts. In any health diplomacy position, you need a health expert who has an understanding of the global context and can then become a diplomat, in that order"* (CORE 4).
Understanding Global Health Instruments, Regulations & Treaties	*"Countries have pandemic funds, but they need to be in place beforehand. The legal frameworks around these kinds of questions are very poorly developed. People, including public health practitioners and Global Health Diplomacy practitioners who are working in these settings, have to have a better understanding of those legal questions and understanding of the legal options to try to deal with them"* (CORE 7). *"We don't have good legal frameworks for the liability questions that come up for legal aspects of pandemics. How do you manage liability around a new vaccine that you're going to give to the general public which has undergone clinical trials, but is still very new, has not had a long time to look at side effects, all these other issues. Who takes the liability?"* (CORE 7).
Performance Frameworks & Capacity Assessments	*"I think there's a pretty significant lack of an ability to really understand our performance framework. The fact that if we're going to put money into things that we want to see results at the end. Sometimes you really do have to say, this isn't working. This agency is not performing its function, let's find someone else. It kind of comes back to that tough love approach, particularly when you're coming from a donor agency. If you're the US, it's not just diplomacy you're often managing, you're providing a lot of the resources, even if you're not managing them. Being insistent on results I think is really important"* (CORE 3).
Training in Intricate Technical Area	*"Often, you would get people that didn't have competencies in diplomatic negotiation, foreign policy, and global governance. Those types of skills include understanding how foreign policy works, how goals are set, and how governments negotiate. So, you get a lot of employees that have no understanding of this because*

4. Critical and Analytical Thinking Knowledge Gaps

This section presents Core GHD actors' expression of knowledge gaps in their

ability to synthesize, analyze, and evaluate information objectively and logically to make

informed and sound decisions.

For one Core GHD actor, GHD actors lacked awareness of the underlying principles of

diagnostic and prevention measures, the science behind vaccine development, and the

limitations of scientific data. They also emphasized GHD actors' ability to negotiate and

make necessary trade-offs, even in the absence of complete information:

*"A lot of people really don't understand infection, prevention, and control. They
don't understand how vaccines work. They don't understand the strengths or the
limitations. They don't understand the whole concept of adverse events and how
they're measured, how they're tracked, and how, in public health, you sometimes
have to make real trade-offs. [There are] some population health questions that
are simply unanswerable, and it will take weeks/months to get the data. They
don't understand that sometimes the data can be wrong. You could actually get
good data, do a thorough analysis, and come up with an entirely reasonable
practical interpretation. And then in a year's time, you could discover that is
completely and utterly wrong. And that's not because of a failure of
understanding, or a failure of performance, or negligence, or malice, or anything
else. It's just that's the way science works"* (CORE 6).

Another Core GHD actor participant also stated that GHD actors should be deeply acquainted and informed about ongoing and emerging situations within their portfolios to allow them to make informed assessments and decisions at short notice if they want to be perceived as competent:

> *"And you need to be versed on what happens, so when something new happens, and you have to pivot from whatever is the situation to what you're gonna be handling, you understand it from the get-go. These are mostly the legal issues that are very tied to the regulatory issues [like] understanding the concept of emergency use authorization. Like, why can't I donate this? Because they're under an emergency situation in my country. Understand the host country's legal and regulatory capabilities, or lack thereof, to import donations during emergencies. That's what can jeopardize your role as an expert on global health security and Global Health Diplomacy if you're not prepared"* (CORE 4).

The same Core GHD actor reiterated how critical it was for experienced health experts to take the lead in GHD efforts, especially during health emergencies. They mentioned that besides having the required knowledge, skills, and competencies, their expertise helps increase trust and credibility among their foreign counterparts:

> *"I know this is very controversial, but I definitely think that any Global Health Diplomacy effort has to be run by the health sector. I feel very strongly about that. I joined the government in [year redacted] at a time when all the plans for pandemic preparedness were saying that in the event of a pandemic, the State Department would take the lead, and H1N1 came, and the State Department had no clue about what to do, neither USAID, you know. It's one thing to work in developing countries having grants and cooperative agreements or donating basic medicines or supplies,. The other is to manage the whole pandemic when you have to work at that interface of the domestic needs and the international needs when the supplies and the vaccine stockpiles and everything belongs to HHS [NIH, FDA, ASPER, Office of Global Affairs]"* (CORE 4).

5. **Practical or Practice-Based Knowledge Gaps**

This section presents Core GHD actors' expression of technical knowledge gaps while practicing Global Health Diplomacy. Core GHD respondents pointed out GHD actors' lack of real-world experience, lack of understanding of the US emergency response, how to mobilize resources to respond to emergencies, and the lack of

knowledge on how to implement lockdowns, amongst other gaps.

Practical or Real-World Global Health Diplomacy Experience

While discussing this theme, one Core GHD actor reemphasized how GHD

actors' lack of practical, cross-cultural field experience hampered their ability to

understand the situational contexts or populations whose interests they may be

representing during multilateral negotiations. For another respondent within this group,

adequately planning for the turnover of GHD actors or key personnel helped facilitate a

proper handover to mitigate the loss of information and institutional knowledge by

facilitating the transfer of information from outgoing to incoming staff:

> *"That's why overlap from staff is really important. That's why having people on
> the ground who can work in this environment is important. If you work inside an
> Embassy, people will help you and show you how the system works. And
> generally, you know CDC, NIH, and FDA send smart people out that figure this
> stuff out but imagine if we were able to train them in these competencies"* (CORE
> 2).

Understanding the US Emergency Response System

One Core GHD actor expressed how crucial it was that GHD actors, especially

those representing US interests, understand the US emergency response system and the

roles and responsibilities of each federal agency within the system. They insisted that

GHD actors also familiarize themselves with the guidelines and restrictions around the

movement and distribution of emergency supplies:

> *"In a pandemic and or a massive outbreak like Ebola, you are going to be facing
> all the issues of international donations of resources, deployment of personnel,
> emergency medical teams, epidemiological emergency teams, vaccines, antivirals,
> and all the ancillary supplies for the development of diagnostics. So, you need to
> understand the emergency response system of the United States and what the
> domestic limitations and opportunities are. There are a lot of laws that regulate
> what you can donate, who can donate, and when you can donate. In the midst of
> overseeing all the donations and stockpiles, there's also all the domestic demand,*

which they tell you is American taxpayers' money, so it's for the taxpayer. Then you have the pressure from the countries around the world, from international organizations saying, well, this is a pandemic, if we don't stop it everywhere, we don't stop it anywhere" (CORE 4).

The same Core GHD actor further acknowledged the global community's duty toward controlling the spread of infectious disease at the source, as they noted that total containment is hardly feasible:

> *"As long as you keep having disease somewhere, you're always gonna be risking having the disease entering your country and spreading everywhere. So, there are legal, regulatory, logistical, and funding barriers to doing this, and it's very important to understand the mechanisms. Sometimes, the policies changed from administration to administration, and you have to restart the novel"* (CORE 4)

Understanding Donor Requirements and Financial Accountability

One Core GHD actor articulated GHD actors' deficiencies in understanding financial accountability or results frameworks designed to ensure that human and material resources invested produce designated outcomes. They specifically called out the lack of accountability within some UN systems that stemmed from the lack of knowledge of financial planning or programming, especially in multi-year programs:

> *"When you're talking about programming a lot of money, there is the accountability and the ability to really be rigorous in how you're programming that money year to year. I've often been dumbfounded at colleagues looking at performance metrics and just saying, 'Okay, yeah, this looks fine,' without really understanding what they mean. I think that's actually a pretty consistent problem. I think there is often very poor accountability in a lot of the UN agencies. UNICEF is a bit of an exception because they are based entirely on voluntary contributions, so they really need to be results-focused, but that is just not how most of the other UN agencies operate"* (CORE 3).

Conducting Lockdowns and Social Distancing Measures

For one Core GHD actor, a significant challenge that GHD actors and policymakers faced was a lack of understanding of how to implement non-pharmaceutical measures such as lockdown procedures or stay-at-home orders without completely disrupting economic activities. They also mentioned the challenge that came

with ascertaining whether lockdowns were effective and, if so, to what extent:

> *"One of the things that continues to be hotly debated both, I know, at the domestic level, but also here [Geneva]as well, is in terms of the non-pharmaceutical measures for control of a pandemic, lockdowns and so forth. And this question comes round and round and round: Do lockdowns work? And, of course, you and I both know if there's a single-sentence answer to the question: Do lockdowns work? The answer is, of course, it depends. It depends on the pathogen. It depends on the circumstance. It depends on the population. It depends on what you mean by working. If you do a lockdown, it depends on what lockdown means; certain measures will have predictable effects. Will those effects have the magnitude that you think they will, and will they have secondary effects that are unpredictable? And will they actually be 'the right policy or not'? The answer to those questions is that it depends, and people who are not familiar with public health or clinical medicine get deeply uncomfortable with this"* (CORE 6).

6. **Learning Knowledge Gaps**

This section presents Core GHD actors' expressions of technical knowledge gaps

in the processes through which GHD actors acquire knowledge, information, or skills

through previous experience, which leads to positive change that enhances practice.

Participants within this group emphasized the importance of GHD actors learning from

the past to be better prepared for future outbreaks, citing previous events like Ebola, the

Swine flu, the Fukushima nuclear disaster, or the Haiti earthquake. Core GHD actors also

mentioned the challenge GHD actors faced in managing the recent infodemic, rife with

misinformation and disinformation.

Ability to Learn from the Past

Several Core GHD actors expressed the meaningful learning opportunity that

COVID-19 offered them, as well as policy and decision-makers. They recommended that

GHD actors take into consideration infectious disease outbreaks and the likelihood of another pandemic occurring that would warrant them to execute these responsibilities

when the need arose:

> *"I think it's very important that folks who are going to be playing these roles*
> *abroad understand and learn lessons from the big things, from H1N1 to Ebola to*
> *Fukushima to Haiti to COVID, a variety of natural disasters, and that they*
> *become versed with domestic lessons learned and the international lessons*
> *learned because they're going to have to be playing that role"* (CORE 4).

Another Core GHD actor reiterated how the events around the COVID-19 pandemic had

affected every sector, forcing their activities to grind to a halt. They emphasized the need

to ensure Global Health Diplomats are at the discussion table when pertinent

conversations about global security are being had:

> *"What I really fought for with COVID when I had a seat at the table in one of our*
> *large strategic meetings was to remind people; 'No, no, no, stop! In 2020, we shut*
> *down the world, and we didn't shut down the world because of an asteroid. We*
> *didn't shut it down because of a nuclear war. We didn't shut it down because there*
> *was a devastating typhoon. We didn't shut it down because of transnational*
> *criminal networks or because of terrorist events; we shut it down because of a*
> *virus.' And so, you cannot come to conversations about security, about*
> *fundamental international relations, about those kinds of issues and not having*
> *health at the table"* (CORE 7).

Some Core GHD actors expressed concern that any lessons from the recent pandemic

may soon be forgotten, and policymakers may fail to prioritize preparedness measures or

other global health issues that were deferred considering the heightened focus on

COVID-19. They maintained that in order to protect Americans from future and

imminent outbreaks, GHD actors needed to work on strengthening pandemic

preparedness efforts in the rest of the world:

> *"Bureaucracy changes very slowly until it doesn't, until there's an opportunity to*
> *surge forward. And maybe that opportunity is in this post-COVID era, where we*
> *could really make a difference. Because of the challenges of COVID-19 in every*
> *country and around the globe, that's gonna happen again; it's just a matter of*
> *time. And we need to improve our system so that we can mitigate the impact on*
> *humanity. We can help protect America by projecting our public health*
> *competence globally, and without concerted effort in institutions and in the*

*workforce, it's gonna happen again, and we're gonna have the same outcome, the
same struggles. We know how to fix it; it's just getting more dialogue around what
we need to do, what we need to change"* (CORE 2).

Another Core GHD actor commented on the apparent neglect of other global health
issues, such as aging and non-communicable diseases that have a sustained economic
impact on populations and health systems:

> *"I worry that people will forget the lessons of COVID, and I worry that people
> don't really appreciate that these other issues [non-communicable diseases] have
> a bigger economic impact because it's like a dripping faucet. No one really pays
> attention to it, and then demographic changes; aging is not a sickness, aging is
> not a disability, but if you don't have enough people in the middle to feed and take
> care of the people on the other end, that's going to be an economic crisis for
> countries as well"* (CORE 5).

Countering and Managing Mis-and-Disinformation

Core GHD actors highlighted managing mis- and -disinformation as a critical
learning area for GHD actors. Reflecting on the plethora of non-factual information that
flooded media and social media outlets, one Core GHD actor admitted: *"We weren't
ready for the amount of disinformation that happened; we weren't prepared for that"*
(CORE 5).

7. Communication Knowledge Gaps

This section presents Core GHD actors' expression of gaps in knowledge in the
use of various communication formats, such as written, verbal, public speaking, elevator
pitches, and crisis/risk communication, in GHD practice. Participants within this group
highlighted the lack of knowledge on how to access information promptly and how to
communicate risk, particularly in health emergencies.

Access to Information and Knowledge Dissemination

Core GHD actors insisted that knowing how and where to access information is crucial for GHD actors. One respondent within this group shared the benefits of having formal communication channels for US diplomatic missions abroad, which supported the exchange of information and negotiations between US GHD actors and their international counterparts:

> *"We had informal communication channels because the formal communication channels had broken down; they had ended agreements. These MOUs [Memoranda of Understanding] were critical to this regular dialogue because the staff would prepare key topics in advance of the formal leaders' meeting, and we would pretty much know what the other side was going to say; we would know where the red lines were, where to push and where to pull, where we could give and where we couldn't"* (CORE 2).

Communication in Emergencies

Regarding communication in emergencies, one Core GHD actor affirmed that GHD actors must be prepared to communicate during crises and know how to develop a communication plan. However, they also acknowledged the challenges that came with this responsibility and GHD actors knowing how to strike the delicate balance of keeping the population informed without sparking fear, anxiety, or chaos:

> *"And you also need to figure out pretty early on what your communication strategy is going to be so that you can combat bad information because we saw that flourish pretty quickly. Everyone saw what was coming in, and they're like, oh, it's SARS all over again, and that was 20 years ago. It is human nature to deny that the worst is happening, and I think we were all in a state of denial. But at the same time, how do you act on an emerging pandemic in the face of past behavior where we don't want to scare people because that's gonna be a problem?"* (CORE 5).

Understanding Risk and Risk Communication

One Core GHD actor commented on GHD's actors' inability to communicate or convey risk to the public, which they said arose mainly from the actors' lack of knowledge and understanding of how to do so. They further insisted that GHD actors

understand risk as an ongoing process as opposed to having an isolated outlook of the

situation at hand:

> *"As a general rule, people don't understand risk very well. People don't understand risk as a continuum; they understand risk as an absolute or an either-or condition, and we don't do well in communicating that. Probably that's because many of our technical people either don't understand it themselves, or they again don't have that elevator speech, right? They're not good at being able to communicate it. So, understanding the principles around risk and how it can layer on, how it can be based on frequency, dose, or on different contacts, that you can layer on prevention. That it's not an either-or kind of thing"* (CORE 7).

Erosion of Public Trust

Core GHD actors commented on how the lack of understanding of scientific

uncertainty in Public Health practitioners' and policymakers' communications became

increasingly polarizing during the pandemic. One participant within this category noted

that responses that communicated incertitude around the effectiveness of non-

pharmaceutical measures such as social distancing and lockdowns were especially

divisive. They explained the challenge of responding to questions about science or public

health with definitive answers:

> *"People might think you don't know what you are talking about or think you are talking out of both sides of your mouth, and they say they want a simple answer. Well, if I give you a simple answer, it will be wrong. That's also part of diplomacy. You need to have a way to communicate that uncertainty but nevertheless give people something concrete and actionable that they can do. It's hard. It's tough"* (CORE 6).

Another Core GHD actor commented on how the politicization of public health within

the US interfered with the CDC's role during the COVID response, which affected the

institution's credibility as well:

> *"In the US, politics got in the way of CDC doing a good job, and I think the CDC lost its confidence because of what it was going through politically and, because of it, made some big errors"* (CORE 5).

Multistakeholder Global Health Diplomacy Actors' Technical Knowledge Gaps

This section presents Multistakeholder GHD actors' expression of technical

knowledge gaps in the practical or theoretical understanding of Global Health

Diplomacy.

1. **Systemic Gaps**

This section presents Multistakeholder GHD actors' expression of gaps within

public health, political, governance, or regulatory systems that resulted in a sub-optimal

response to the COVID-19 pandemic. Respondents within this group emphasized gaps in

the pandemic preparedness and response efforts, inadequate public health resources and

infrastructure, as well as the lack of public health personnel during the pandemic.

Pandemic Preparedness, Detection, and Response

Some Multistakeholder GHD actors mentioned addressing pandemic

preparedness by strengthening countries' surveillance, diagnostic, and response capacities

as critical for the post-COVID era:

> *"I think having a really clear plan for each country on how to build up
> surveillance, data management, and patient management is hard. We do have that
> in many countries, but again, it's just so hard when you have so many
> stakeholders having different priorities and preferences for different data systems.
> And it takes a long time for these data systems to develop, so that's particularly
> challenging"* (MSTK 3).

Another Multistakeholder GHD actor admitted that while their agency had invested time

and resources in these areas in the past, it has become an even bigger focus post-COVID.

They went further to describe their efforts to ensure more robust surveillance and data

systems were set up around the world to facilitate the rapid detection, containment, and

reporting of infectious disease outbreaks:

> *"So, the work that we do was always in that lane more or less, but now, I think, it
> is more directed to "let's make sure the surveillance systems are in order. Let's*

make sure the data systems are in order so that if someone comes in and they have a fever and it's not the flu, we do a diagnostic, we have an index of suspicion of what could this be? We have places to send the specimen, and we know how to send a specimen, how to report that, and who can help. And all those things need to be in place now. And so, I think a lot of not just the CDC but also WHO, USAID, and many different organizations are working towards that right, which is how to prepare for the next COVID by building systems" (MSTK 7).

One Multistakeholder GHD actor recognized the importance and urgency of strengthening emergency response systems to increase their resiliency against future outbreaks and health security threats. However, the same respondent also noted the challenges these efforts posed as countries were faced with competing priorities, post-pandemic economic recovery, pandemic fatigue, and turnover within political leadership:

"Countries pivoted so dramatically to COVID, and it had a huge economic impact on many countries. And so, getting back to normal is really important from an economic point of view and [also] from a stress point of view. So, keeping in the forefront of your mind that no, no, but we have to be ready for the next thing is challenging when there are many 'now, now' things that people are worried about and don't wanna think about that [COVID] anymore. Or sometimes the political strength behind that kind of work is dependent on someone who's in office today who may not be in office tomorrow and so doesn't care as much. So, it's challenging to keep that momentum, because it's also to prevent and it is hard to measure what you didn't do and what didn't happen, and so it's hard to get people to stay motivated" (MSTK 7).

Public Health Resources and Infrastructure

One Multistakeholder GHD actor stated that the public health sector within the US was underfunded, which they said translated to low remuneration for public health practitioners, personnel burnout, lack of modern technology, and insufficient resources for an adequate pandemic response. They also mentioned the high turnover from personnel burnout during the pandemic:

"We haven't put a lot of resources into the payment stream. To bring those critical skill sets, you have to have the technology on board. At the strategic level, you may have all of the technological advances, but when you start getting down to the trenches, when you start getting down to rural Alabama or Georgia, Tennessee, a lot of those public health departments do not have the technical

resources or human resources, because they do not have the money to attract them. So, we have to infuse the resources from the top down. Also, the local departments need to advertise and get in the business of really speaking about the things that they're doing and what they could have done more of had they had additional resources to do that" (MSTK 2).

Human Resource or Staffing Gaps

For several Multistakeholder GHD actors, COVID-19 exposed existing human resource gaps. They added that the difficulty of filling those gaps in an emergency context impeded GHD actors' and their counterparts' ability to respond to the pandemic effectively, particularly noting the specific lack of technical expertise around COVID-19 vaccination:

> *"Staffing was a real challenge during COVID; having the right staff with the appropriate skills was hard. But it's also about being able to cross-train people because you can't rely on that one staff member who really has deep knowledge of a topic area or even of a technical area; you need to make sure you have that kind of breath across the organization so that you can all respond to something like, let's say Anthrax, especially when we looked at expertise related to immunization. But really, in any technical area, having people cross-trained and mentorship is really important"* (MSTK 3).

Data and Essential Resources Gaps

More than half of the Multistakeholder GHD respondents in this group expressed GHD actors' inability to access data and essential resources and supplies promptly, such as PPE and diagnostic tests, which they said were essential for the pandemic response. One Multistakeholder GHD actor also highlighted the lack of modern and portable technology for contact-tracing, as well as the time it took for the data to be made available, which could sometimes be from two days prior:

> *"The [contact tracing] technology has to be portable, and that costs, right? Also, a lot of the data that we were using, at least from my standpoint, sometimes could be a day or two days old. So, how do you compare trends? I had to remind folks that the data that I'm presenting to you was taken off the mainframe yesterday"* (MSTK 2).

2. **Interpersonal Gaps**

This section presents Multistakeholder GHD actors' expression of knowledge

gaps in traits and abilities that GHD actors require for harmonious interactions with one's

team and with others from diverse cultural backgrounds, facilitating the building and

fostering of relationships.

Collaboration and Teamwork

Reflecting on some challenges in interpersonal interactions during the pandemic,

one Multistakeholder GHD actor highlighted some challenges in team cohesion that

negatively impacted their overall performance at the time:

> *"Definitely, teamwork is critical, and in that specific job, we struggled as a team*
> *in the beginning, and it got to a point where I was like, hey, let's take some time;*
> *we need to get it together because people's lives and people's health to rely on*
> *what we're doing"* (MSTK 4).

3. **Technical, Intricate, or Expert Area Knowledge Gaps**

Multistakeholder GHD actors expressed several gaps in GHD practice, displayed

by a lack of theoretical or practical understanding of several intricate technical areas.

Some of these gaps included a lack of knowledge in vaccines, diagnostics and

therapeutics, epidemiology and statistics, and informatics and web technology. These

technical knowledge gaps are presented in the table below:

Table 16

Multistakeholder GHD Actors' Expression of Technical Knowledge Gaps

Technical Knowledge Gap	Multistakeholder GHD Actor Excerpt
Training in Intricate Technical Area	*"Being trained and doffed on procedures, being trained on how to interact with irate passengers. Being trained on certain questions, even though we won't know everything and have the answer for everything, but having been trained to have some sort of answer is really important for communicating things appropriately, scientifically, and accurately. Training is important, and it shouldn't be a one-time thing. It should be*

	ongoing; we should be constantly trained as information changes" (MSTK 4).
Knowledge of Vaccines, Diagnostics & Therapeutics	*"Well, I brought one example of this 'lumping things together' in terms of whether we are talking drugs, vaccines, PPE, or diagnostics. And all of these things will have different processes in terms of how they are developed and the science behind them, and also how they're produced and how they are kept and all of these other things that come later. I mean a simple example of the fact knowing that different vaccines need different kinds of cold chain." (MSTK 6).* *"I think that the key knowledge gap was just the testing; being able to explain to individuals what's the difference between PCR, rapid antigen, rapid PCR, all those different tests. And then the home tests and being able to explain why we can't use the results from this. I feel like that was the most prominent question. And a lot of times we were unprepared to answer those kinds of questions, so we would deflect and kind of circumvent our answers and try to avoid them. But I think that was only because we were not specifically trained on how to answer those questions" (MSTK 4).*
Epidemiology and Statistics	*"Maybe one thing that everybody could use a refresher course on is some of the epidemiological implications, but maybe that's my bias as an epidemiologist" (MSTK 5).* *"Being abreast of incidence rates, prevalence rates, even knowing the difference, just having those Epi statistics with us, not just in a way that we understand it, but also providing that information in a way that the population we were working with can understand it because not everyone's going to understand incidence rates" (MSTK 4).*
Informatics/ Web Technology	*"Any type of technology has a short shelf life, and you have to think about the generational gap. You have folks who can't connect to Zoom. Also, for folks coming out of school programs, they have to understand that they're walking into a multi-component generational setting" (MSTK 2)*

4. Practical or Practice-Based Knowledge Gaps

This section presents Multistakeholder GHD actors' expression of GHD actors' technical knowledge gaps while practicing Global Health Diplomacy. Respondents noted leadership challenges that arose from a lack of health-related technical expertise.

Leadership

Reflecting on the role of leadership in GHD, one Multistakeholder GHD actor talked about how the absence of strong leadership and clear direction posed challenges within their teams during the COVID-19 response:

> *"We were literally trying to figure it out on our own [at the quarantine station], and I don't know if leadership is necessarily a technical skill, but definitely having and placing specific leaders to lead teams was something that could have been helpful for us"* (MSTK 4).

Diplomacy for "wrong or unaltruistic" reasons

While Multistakeholder GHD actors insisted that GHD actors acquire the required *"knowledge of the Global Health Diplomacy field overall,"* one respondent within this group cautioned that not all GHD actors practice Global Health Diplomacy for altruistic reasons:

> *"A lot of the countries will use diplomacy to disrupt other countries. Other countries will not have a straightforward diplomacy process simply because they are not a democracy. Their line of decision-making is completely different, and the process is completely different, not better or worse. But it's different. So, you look at the world where maybe only 20% of people live in what we would call a democracy, which means that 80% do not. Hence, all the diplomatic processes in the country may or may not always subscribe to the generalization that we're talking about here"* (MSTK 6).

5. Learning Knowledge Gaps

This section presents Multistakeholder GHD actors' expression of technical knowledge gaps in the processes through which GHD actors acquire knowledge, information, or skills through a previous experience that leads to positive change that enhances practice. Participants asserted the importance of GHD actors learning from past events as well as being willing to learn amid the changing scope and demands of their roles.

Ability to Learn from the Past

Some Multistakeholder GHD actors affirmed that learning lessons and recommendations from the COVID-19 pandemic and previous global health emergencies can inform current and future pandemic preparedness measures. For one Multistakeholder GHD actor, in addition to doing their pre-deployment research, GHD actors should seek out just-in-time training to prepare them for the roles to which they will be assigned:

> *"Before we [US GHD actors] go into these countries, it would be great if we had the research and training readily available and a one-pager or two-pager about things we should be thinking about. You would think that COVID has taught us a lesson, but what I've also learned is we forget. That's why we keep repeating a lot of these things [mistakes]" (MSTK 2).*

On-the-job Learning

Multistakeholder GHD actors said GHD actors should be willing and able to acquire new technical knowledge as the needs arise. One respondent within this group argued that being a Global Health Diplomat did not require profound technical expertise as GHD actors were often confronted with myriads of issues that require learning on the job:

> *"If someone wants to have a State Department career with a focus on health diplomacy, they don't really need deep technical expertise. I mean, they have to learn it as they go. So obviously, you should have Health 101 and learn about the global burden of disease and general knowledge. But it's such a broad field. Some people, knowing their limitations, can learn what a lab leak versus bioengineered versus natural emergence of an infection means. And what's the data from the Wuhan fish markets? Are they keeping their eyes wide open and not being swayed by political arguments or misinformation? They didn't need to have a lot of background knowledge to be able to learn about that" (MSTK 5).*

The same Multistakeholder GHD actor emphasized the need for GHD actors with scientific and health expertise to learn and develop their communication and diplomacy skills, which are central to their roles, even if they said many of them were largely unaware of this. The respondent also recommended a hybrid approach to training GHD

actors that allowed for in-person and virtual participation:

> *"A lot of CDC and NIH staff are like, 'Oh, we're scientists, we don't even do communications, never mind diplomacy.' And they really need to learn that, if they don't think they do it, they're just doing it really badly because they are doing it [Global Health Diplomacy], whether they know it or not. Being in Washington, DC, [for training] will be easier with PEPFAR, State Department, NIH, and folks here, but with virtual learning or people coming from Atlanta, that could also have the CDC audience"* (MSTK 5).

6. **Communication Knowledge Gaps**

This section presents Multistakeholder GHD actors' expression of gaps in

knowledge on the use of various communication formats, such as written, verbal, public

speaking, elevator pitches, and crisis/risk communication, in GHD practice. Participants

highlighted the lack of knowledge of foreign languages, in addition to knowing how to

communicate in emergencies.

Communication in Emergencies

Multistakeholder GHD actor stated that trust is essential when communicating

during emergencies, and clear and accurate communication helps establish credibility.

One participant within this group vocalized how the lack of training on how to represent

the US government appropriately made them appear untrustworthy, which they said also

impacted the United States' credibility:

> *"With the issue of public trust and not being credible as government officials, that would have been something we should have been trained on. We were the face of the [US] government at that point, even if we didn't want to believe it. We were representing the government and what the government wanted. So, I think that broke a lot of trust because we were not able to be a good, credible face"* (MSTK 4).

Foreign Language Gaps

While discussing the relevance of foreign languages, one Multistakeholder GHD actor reflected on how the lack of knowledge of the Spanish language posed a communication barrier between their team and international passengers who neither understood nor spoke English:

> *"I know I mentioned language multiple times, but language skills, whether it means hiring specific translators or just having translators available. They gave us a phone hotline to call [for translation services], and no one was ever available. So, we didn't even use that"* (MSTK 4).

Informal Global Health Diplomacy Actors' Technical Knowledge Gaps

This section presents Informal GHD actors' expression of technical knowledge gaps in the practical or theoretical understanding of Global Health Diplomacy. These gaps have been categorized into Systemic, Interpersonal, Technical, Practical or Practice-Based, Critical and Analytical Thinking, Learning, and Communication knowledge gaps.

1. **Systemic Gaps**

This section presents Informal GHD actors' expression of gaps within public health, political, governance, or regulatory systems that resulted in a sub-optimal response to the COVID-19 pandemic. Respondents in this group emphasized gaps in the pandemic preparedness and response efforts, the lack of data access and essential supplies such as PPE, inadequate public health resources and infrastructure, and the lack of public health personnel during the pandemic.

Pandemic Preparedness, Detection, and Response

While discussing pandemic preparedness gaps, a third of Informal GHD actors reflected on specific areas that countries had failed to prioritize, making them largely unprepared for the COVID-19 pandemic. One participant within this group called out countries' non-adherence to previous efforts and recommendations to strengthen the

global health security infrastructure:

> *"The gaps in terms of pandemic prevention, detection, and response have been identified through the Global Health Security Agenda and the Joint External Evaluations. Too little attention is paid, even though there is a very large agreement amongst over 90 countries and bodies. There is a structure of being able to prevent, detect, and respond to pandemics, and that receives very short strip. Instead, the world seems to be occupied with developing a pandemic treaty, and I'll be an outlier, probably in saying this, but that's not the route to strengthen the international community's ability to be more effective at responding to future pandemics"* (INFML 5).

Another Informal GHD actor commented on the domino effect that the US' lack of

preparedness had on the rest of the world:

> *"We put our money in our diplomatic emphasis elsewhere; that's not even controversial; that's been analyzed and identified; and paid a huge price. Again, that's a choice. We chose to prioritize HIV/AIDS in developing countries, Global Fund, Malaria, TB, and HIV/AIDS. Wonderful things happened. I'm not trying to be critical of those programs, but in terms of our interests, we didn't protect ourselves from a pandemic. And because we weren't ready, the collateral damage on the rest of the world was more than it needed to be. So, it's not just that we were hurt, but the fact that we weren't ready created all of the problems, and the damage was globalized because we're a great power, just like in the great recession that started in the US"* (INFML 2).

The same Informal GHD actor also highlighted the US' failings in addressing its top two

foreign policy issues:

> *"We never got our act together on climate change, which is the biggest chronic threat to our people's health, our economy, our national security. So, if we go back to just basic foreign policy interest; We failed to deal with the two biggest acute and chronic threats to our foreign policy interests. So, we might have done great diplomacy on some other issues, I don't wanna take those down, but we weren't focused on what was supposed to be according to the way that we say we think about these top issues"* (INFML 2).

Furthermore, the Informal GHD actor further recognized the impact of the US'

inadequacies on its foreign policy, as well as the potential loss of credibility in the eyes of

the rest of the world:

"CFR [The Council on Foreign Relations] has this whole Renewing America Initiative, which is looking at how we have neglected our homeland, and that's having foreign policy consequences. Now, that's not diplomacy in the sense that you and I are talking about it now, but it affects the credibility of what you do diplomatically. If I'm other countries, I'm looking at the US, with all the news stories that have been coming out about life expectancies in the US. I'm just like, why should we listen to them? We listen to them because they have money, which we (US) don't, right? They listen because we're still powerful. Well, we're in a different context here. I'm not happy to say that, but triage, right? Prioritizations: where are we gonna put scarce resources? I think the demands from other countries on the climate change issues, we cannot escape that going forward. That's happening right now in COP 28. It's here, it's now, we don't have a plan" (INFML 2).

Another Informal GHD actor highlighted the stark disparities and capacity gaps between

countries that had access to essential pandemic supplies and how soon they had access:

"There's a lot of problems and issues with equity and resource mobilization in terms of when you're talking about vaccines or access to vaccines. Communication did contribute to some of those gaps, too. So, there are gaps in communication, in the workforce, in the provision of resources, in the provision of vaccines, gaps in the dissemination of information in terms of how to prevent or protect oneself and prevent the transmission of COVID-19. On the diagnostic side, the capacity in the country was another knowledge gap because there's a lot of information that needs to be disseminated to the healthcare providers and first responders, the ability to actually have adequate PPE available. All of those capacity gaps, knowledge gaps, and resource gaps were there in terms of building up an adequate response" (INFML 6).

The same Informal GHD actor elaborated on other drivers of vaccine inequity. They

asserted vaccine inequity stemmed mainly from the private sector's hold on intellectual

property rights to vaccine production, which they said made them unaffordable and

inaccessible primarily to low and middle-income countries at the heart of the pandemic

when they needed it most:

"[Failure] to share the vaccine adequately and to diversify. We should have known this in Ebola to be able to have diversified production facilities around the world, particularly in LMICs. Governments should not assert when they are giving money to the private sector, but they should have negotiated an agreement where whatever they discover would be a public good and public property. But it

is a situation where the private sector gets everything or can run away with it, although public funds were distributed. So, I think this is a failure to share the intellectual property, to negotiate the funding agreement initially, so it became a public good, to strengthen the production capacity in low resource settings, in particular production facilities that were already identified, but were never focused on, to be able to ensure that there was more equitable distribution of that" (INFML 5).

Public Health Resources and Infrastructure

With regard to the lack of public health resources and infrastructure, one Informal

GHD actor compared the current state of US public health departments to how they were

almost three decades ago:

> *"When I first started doing this in 1995, one of the big complaints from domestic public health agencies was communication, and this was the time when the Internet was already coming on stream. They were still sending stuff back and forth by faxes! What do we hear during the COVID? The same complaint! Again, this goes to the lack of preparation; we didn't take our own public health seriously enough. So, we have a lot of domestic repair to be done. Doing that repair is important to being credible in our foreign policy. And this is true across lots of issue areas, not just health"* (INFML 2).

Data and Essential Resource Gaps

While reflecting on insufficiencies in data availability and access to essential

resources, another Informal GHD actor hailed the US' federal efforts to fast-track vaccine

development and distribution through Operation Warp Speed as a key success of the

Trump Administration's pandemic response:

> *"I think to the credit of President Trump being able to invest rapidly in the development and investment in a vaccine was critically important. But for those countries that had domestic production, capacity to produce the vaccine, to produce the PPE that was necessary and to have a rapid ability to produce diagnostics like testing tech kits that were reliable was really important. So, I think that those combination of things before a vaccine came on board was really important, and that solutions are titrated according to the local situation cause it's never a one-size fits all as we know"* (INFML 5).

The same Informal GHD actor further noted the lack of quality control in the production of personal protective equipment that resulted in the manufacture and sale of sub-standard commodities like face masks and PPE, as well as vaccine hoarding:

> *"There wasn't adequate distribution and capacity to scale up the production of PPE, nor was there a willingness to actually invest in the capacity of other sites around the world, particularly LMICs, to produce PPE. And, of course, vaccine hoarding that happened in countries like Canada and others, including here in the United States, was really shameful in an appalling way. Despite the fact that people have been talking about equity for a long time, they really showed how much equity really means when the rubber meets the road, and it didn't"* (INFML 5).

2. **Technical, Intricate, or Expert Area Knowledge Gaps**

Informal GHD actors expressed various gaps in GHD practice, displayed by a lack of theoretical or practical understanding of several intricate technical areas. One respondent within this group asserted that identifying technical knowledge gaps would depend on what the GHD actor was asked to do and what human and material resources they had at their disposal for addressing these gaps. Other participants mentioned the knowledge of capacity and performance, informatics and web technology, and an understanding of global health instruments, regulations, and treaties, captured in the table below:

Table 17

Informal GHD Actors' Expression of Technical Knowledge Gaps in GHD Practice

Technical Knowledge Gap	Informal GHD Actor Excerpt
Performance Frameworks & Capacity Assessments	*"Let's look at them from the standpoint of assessments; some of the assessments that the WHO might have done from the Joint External Evaluation; I don't know as to how reflective they were off the actual capacities on the ground. Maybe not so much in certain countries, and maybe close in other countries; it depends on how truthful the countries were and how the evaluations were done. And that's something to be looked at. So, obviously, there's a knowledge gap"* (INFML 6).
Informatics/ Web Technology	*"Being comfortable with communication channels like Zoom or Microsoft Teams and also, not being so rigid [about which channel to use], being open to the different channels of*

	communication depending on the individual's request is really important" (INFML 7).
	"I didn't know anything about Microsoft Power BI, but I definitely think that's a wonderful tool to visualize your data, and the team and I had to learn how to use that. I do think images and graphs tell a story. And being comfortable with utilizing that to showcase [the data to] the Ministry of Health or other stakeholders was very important" (INFML 7).
Training in Intricate Technical Area	*"How do you communicate effectively across multiple different stakeholders and avenues throughout an emergency in order to make effective policy decisions and communications out to the population? And then systems thinking which kind of ties into the public health ethics and emergency preparedness and One Health, because I feel like One Health really pulls in all of the areas of public health that could lead to a potential disaster or emergency. Both naturally, man-made, or otherwise. The knowledge that encompasses underneath each of those skill families are what our Global Health Diplomacy folks need and are definitely lacking now. And it's not built into their profession or their educational training to be ready to do all of those skills"* (INFML 4).
	"Certainly, you have to have a knowledge of food production, sanitation, and hygiene, which are generally not taught in schools of public health. That's why I'm advocating for a One Health approach, because maybe the subjects that are being taught were of use in the twentieth century, but we're dealing with very different issues in the twenty-first century that require different knowledge sets." (INFML 3).
	"I usually come at this from a socio-ecological model [of health] when you're looking at a theory because it starts with a person and their community, and that circle goes outward. And that will help you plan better when you really understand that socio-ecologic model because it's not based on just the individual. Let's say, in a pandemic or any type of emergency, who are the actors that would play a role in this? And if we go to the global scale, we would take it to, how would the WHO fit in this? How would the UN fit into this? How would individual countries? How would we deal with low and middle-income countries? Because they always suffer the most when things happen globally, and we have the hoarders like the United States, Russia, and China, who don't necessarily hold their end of the bargain unless sometimes it's to their benefit" (INFML 1)
	"I'd say the biggest one for emergency preparedness is even just risk management and communications; how do you navigate that? Policy and advocacy and I feel that technical gap is so big that I can't even frame it into one sentence. We, as practitioners, are not taught anything political, and I think a benefit of sorts to our field is that we've tried to be apolitical. But because of that, we have distanced ourselves so much from politics that we don't actually know how to navigate the system to push forward policies and laws that would benefit our field at all. What do the

	global, multinational, multilateral governmental structures look like, and how do you interject into that to advocate for policies and change" (INFML 4).
Understanding Global Health Instruments, Regulations & Treaties	*"This is a new space for me; there's definitely a lot of guidelines that the World Health Organization has developed. And so, we all needed to get up to speed on that, specifically on the best therapeutics to use to address COVID-19. We knew that we wanted to implement therapeutics into our project, but we didn't know which ones to tap into. So, we definitely had to refer to WHO for that, even with the rapid testing diagnostics. I think that there's a lot of knowledge gaps around laboratories like the PCR and utilization of the PCR versus utilization of rapid testing. And so, we had to refer to ASLM [African Society of Laboratory Medicine]. There are resources out there; it's just knowing where they are and being able to tap into that and adapt it for your own context"* (INFML 7).

3. Critical and Analytical Thinking Knowledge Gaps

About half of the Informal GHD actors recognized the importance of GHD actors'

ability to analyze, evaluate, and synthesize information objectively for logical decisions.

One Informal GHD actor reflected on GHD actors' and public health professionals' lack

of knowledge of public health ethics frameworks and how these are utilized at the

individual, community, and population levels:

> *"There is a clear distinction between an individual medical decision and a population-level ethical consideration. And I think the result that we've seen is because of not having a clear framework for public health ethics. We saw much more resistance to some of the decisions that were being made based on COVID and pushback on, say, vaccines or policies that are implemented, like masking. Because we really tried to apply population-level policy when everything, especially in our Western culture, not necessarily in other cultures, is very individualistic. There's going to be a trickle-down effect because they didn't systematically think about the implications of this policy in this cultural setting. And so, the knowledge of individual versus population level variables, factors and how you would navigate those in order to develop a policy and then communicate that policy out at large. "* (INFML 4).

Regarding the challenges around vaccines, availability, accessibility, and affordability,

one Informal GHD actor mentioned that GHD actors *"did not have a good understanding of the limitations of their own governments when it comes to vaccine awareness and what*

to do with the public" (INFML 1).

Another Informal GHD actor stressed the need for governments to have negotiated to

ensure the COVID-19 vaccine becomes a public good, for everyone's benefit: :

> *"Governments needed, in my view, to say we're going to invest in this money in your private sector to help us to develop these vaccines and therapeutics. But the flip side of that is whatever you discover is going to be a public good, and it's going to be owned by the people. And we are going to take that IP and that discovery and share wherever we want. So, you wouldn't have to go through the intellectual property challenges that were thrown up for the private sector to make more money in the midst of a crisis"* (INFML 5).

One Informal GHD actor noted the lack of systems thinking, which they said resulted in

an isolationist approach to dealing with global health issues, instead of examining the

entire system and its components. They upheld the One Health approach as being integral

to pandemic preparedness and response efforts:

> *"I feel like some folks, even in the Public Health sphere, aren't aware of what One Health really is and the implications that could have across all of our different sectors. Having that knowledge of who the actors are would be relevant to understanding One Health. If and when another infectious disease pandemic happens, those are the stakeholders and entities and actors that are going to be maybe a little bit ahead of the game because they've been tracking things, they've been up to date, but not all global health practitioners are, and so making sure that there is that clear understanding and awareness of who even tracks these types of activities at large? And then how do we bring it all together and synthesize it into a more global perspective across all of our different sectors since we seem to be a very siloed industry?* (INFML 4).

4. **Practical or Practice-Based Knowledge Gaps**

This section presents Informal GHD actors' expression of GHD actors' technical

knowledge gaps while practicing Global Health Diplomacy. Respondents discussed GHD

actors' knowledge gaps across several domains, including the lack of understanding of

the present geopolitical landscape, a lack of understanding of the US emergency response

and how to appropriately leverage the community in emergency response efforts.

Community Engagement and Community Mobilization

Reflecting on the role of the community in emergencies, a few Informal GHD

actors shared their perspectives on the need and benefits of actively involving community

members in pandemic preparedness and response efforts. One participant recounted:

> *"When we think about Global Health Diplomacy, we talk about NGOs; we don't
> talk about the community, yet they're integral to It. I think, in a post-COVID era,
> it's important to still tap the community to understand the residual effects of
> COVID-19. And what do they think we could improve on in terms of assistance in
> a future pandemic learning from a past one"* (INFML 7).

The same participant further asserted the role of religious leaders and Community Health

Volunteers as a gateway into communities:

> *"In all 3 of our countries, we utilized religious leaders. I feel as though a lot of
> entities forget about them, but they have a lot of influence on behavior change
> and they have a lot of weight. Community Health Volunteers as well. Kenya
> recently changed their name to Community Health Promoters, and in Zimbabwe,
> they're called Community Health Promoters because they are a cadre, and they
> do get paid, not a lot, but they get paid. So, it is important to see that their time is
> valuable and necessary for the fight against any future pandemic"* (INFML 7).

Understanding of Global Health Diplomacy Stakeholders

While discussing the relevance of GHD stakeholders, another Informal GHD

actor vocalized the importance for GHD actors knowing how to conduct a stakeholder

analysis to ascertain who the key stakeholders were, their roles, and the resources they

had at their disposal:

> *"You really need to have a good idea of who your partners are so that if you are
> setting up mass anything, you know who your go-to people with the knowledge
> and background to be able to do it. There's no way for even a Global Health
> Diplomat to know everything. Still, if you're connected, you will get what you
> need from your community partners or other agencies, whether it be
> governmental or non-governmental agencies. I'll give you an example: setting up
> mass vaccination and testing required by multisectoral agencies. You had to
> recruit people to do it, so you have to tap into your community leaders to get the
> word out. However, setting up those mass vaccination testing clinics required the
> police department, the fire department, and a whole variety of folks outside of our*

health department to implement it. So, those are some of the skills that I knew other people had because you just can't do it yourself. Where you don't have the skill set internally, you must be able to lean on others and know where to go" (INFML 1).

Understanding Politics and the Geopolitical Landscape

Looking back at the early days of the pandemic, one Informal GHD actor called

for GHD actors to evaluate why some countries fared better in their efforts to control the

spread of the pandemic compared to others with seemingly greater resources and more

robust response capacity:

> *"I think that the larger problem was a failure to understand politics. If you look at what worked and what didn't work in those countries, whether it was Hong Kong, Taiwan, Japan, or South Korea, that were doing a good job early in the pandemic before the mRNA vaccine was available. Understanding why that was really important because a lot of the factors that made them successful were based on politics. Conversely, why countries such as the United Kingdom, the United States, and others that were identified from scientific assessments to be very well prepared for future pandemics before the pandemic started failed, and they failed largely because of politics and culture. And the culture I'm talking about is the relationship between the public and politicians, trust issues that are built up over generations, and individual characteristics of populations that were really important in being able to identify why certain populations behaved in certain ways, and others didn't. A lot of that was embedded in the culture of countries for good and for ill. But the individualistic cultures, of course, do worse than those that have a collective mentality"* (INFML 5).

The same Informal GHD actor also reflected on the influence of politics and political will

on the implementation of global health policies or interventions:

> *"I think some of the technical solutions are often not that complicated, but for political reasons, they're not addressed. So, a Global Health Diplomacy actor needs to really understand why that's not happening and understand what moves politicians and political actors in the global health community. We're looking for technical and scientific solutions for problems that first need political solutions to address* (INFML 5).

One Informal GHD actor also questioned how prominent the US influence in the global

health arena might be, considering the diminishing interest and support from the

American people. They conveyed that the US no longer has the resources it did 20 years

ago to invest in global health initiatives, especially not at a time when its citizens were

demanding greater accountability from their government following the pitfalls of the

COVID-19 pandemic:

> *"To me, what's interesting is the way in which the US is gonna have to change the way that it does health diplomacy. We were always willing to listen to what African countries wanted. I mean HIV/AIDS; we forget that was the worst pandemic in human history once upon a time. So yeah, PEPFAR was responsive to what African countries wanted and needed. That conversation is much harder today, not just because of COVID, but certainly because of COVID. If they wanted more autonomy and more health sovereignty, how can we help? What does that mean for our foreign policy in the health space? There's this notion that what we [the US] did 20 years ago, we can do again today, no! People don't understand when I say this: the US has no money. Even if Congress appropriates it, we have no money, so we have to borrow it. And that reality isn't sinking in"* (INFML 2).

The same participant went further to explain how geopolitics and foreseeable changes to

the US' role within the global health arena might influence foreign policy priorities,

global health funding, potentially redefining key players in the global health arena:

> *"I think this is a huge problem; if you can't rely on the credibility of the United States, then how do British, South African, and Brazilian foreign policymakers and diplomats look at global health? That's a new world. Even if we didn't like everything the Americans did, they stepped up, they put big money into this, they threw their weight around. Yeah, we complained about it, but if they're not gonna do that anymore, what do we do? I think exploring some ways other countries think about foreign policy, diplomacy, and health is fascinating because the burden will fall on them. We are approaching being utterly hopeless in the US. I don't like saying that, but I can't say with a straight face, well, 'the United States is going to be a global leader,' no! I know there's no political support, no consensus, no bipartisanship, there's no money! That's where Africa, I think is very interesting because they're kind of fed up, right? So, when they think about a new African global health order, how are they thinking about your questions? Same with Brazil. It won't be the G7, G20, the usual suspects* (INFML 2).

Understanding the US Emergency Response System

While discussing the US Emergency Response System, one Informal GHD actor explained the executive branch, states, and local authorities' roles and responsibilities in preventing, protecting against, mitigating, and responding to infectious disease outbreaks:

> *"Keeping disease from coming into the country [US] is a federal responsibility at the ports. And in today's day and age, that's the seaports and the airports. But a public health response is a state and local responsibility. So that makes it the responsibility of the governors and the mayors. If one looks at the 2001 Anthrax scares, we were dealing with bioterrorism. That's a national security issue, and national security is a federal issue. So, when you're dealing with a public health crisis, particularly, say, if it's a bioterrorist attack, then you've got all sorts of different chains of command because it's a national security crisis and a public health crisis. So, you've got all sorts of different leaders, and during Anthrax, nobody knew who was in charge because it was a mess because of the Constitution; it's outdated"* (INFML 3).

Leadership Skills

Reflecting on the importance of leadership skills, the same Informal GHD actor insisted on how the shortfalls of leadership during the pandemic, beginning from the US executive office, led to higher COVID-19 mortality rates:

> *"We lost many lives unnecessarily because of his poor leadership and the failings of his administration. The CDC really bungled it. And we didn't have a functional chain of command; that was messed up too"* (INFML 3).

Conducting Lockdowns and Social Distancing Measures

Informal GHD actors also stated that GHD actors and policymakers faced a dilemma on how best to implement measures to control the spread of the virus at the population level:

> *"Nobody knew how to do the [pandemic] response adequately. Did they need to lock up everybody? Otherwise, the country's economy would suffer a lot, and instead of doing lockdowns, how to do it in a much more systematic [manner such as] smart lockdowns. How to contain the transmission of infection rather than actually shutting everything down. And that actually caused a lot of issues from an economic standpoint for a lot of countries, too"* (INFML 6).

5. **Learning Knowledge Gaps**

This section presents Informal GHD actors' expression of technical knowledge

gaps in the processes through which GHD actors acquire knowledge, information, or

skills through a previous experience that leads to positive change that enhances practice.

Informal GHD actors emphasized the importance of GHD actors learning as they go and

from the past to better equip for handling future emergencies. Respondents within this

group also emphasized the need for GHD actors to learn how to manage mis-and

disinformation.

Ability to Learn from the Past

As Informal GHD actors reflected on crucial learning opportunities, one Informal

GHD actor stated that many adverse effects of the COVID-19 pandemic could have been

circumvented had countries invested in making their health systems more resilient after

the Ebola crisis:

> *"Technically, I think, we still fall down the rabbit hole of failing to actually
> strengthen that which came out of the Ebola outbreak. The gaps were identified
> by the Joint External Evaluations. Even with that, we still see that those low-
> hanging fruits are not necessarily dealt with. If I go back to the Ebola outbreak, a
> failure to build on the investments during a crisis takes place, but there isn't
> adequate thought to be able to use those investments for long-term health systems
> strengthening that can come out of a crisis so that a country can be strengthened
> in the long, long term for future pandemics. That was a failure in the Ebola crisis,
> where so much money was poured into countries that were vulnerable, but it
> wasn't organized properly to make sure that those countries were really
> strengthened in the long term. And that's a real tragedy"* (INFML 5)

Another Informal GHD actor shared a similar perspective, calling for proper capacity

assessments to be done to first identify systemic shortfalls before attempting to address

them:

> *"We need to learn from our deficiencies during the COVID pandemic and what
> those deficiencies were. There might be differing deficiencies for different*

countries, and we need to know how to address them so that they can be well prepared for a future pandemic. Those things need to be taken into account when you are looking at the Global Health Diplomacy post-COVID" (INFML 6)

One Informal GHD actor recommended a more proactive approach to pandemic preparedness and response efforts by leveraging the lessons of the past:

"It can't be 'let's wait around and wait and see.' Monkeypox was a prime example of this. We were slow to respond, but not nearly as slow as we were to respond to COVID-19. So, we did learn something from that. And we did learn during that time that if we don't have the answers, then we have to look outside of the United States for answers. There was no current research related to monkeypox vaccination. So, we really had to look at this one study from 2015. [Being proactive] requires you to be willing to go outside of your comfort zone. You've got to be willing to do research and come up with factual information and not guess that stuff because it erodes the trust that the public will have" (INFML 1).

Another Informal GHD actor noted that because the majority of response efforts were directly tied to COVID-19 relief funding, once the funding ran out, pandemic preparedness and response efforts were also halted, as countries had not apportioned funding reserves to continue supporting preventive measures.

On-the-Job Learning

While discussing GHD actors' ability to learn, one Informal GHD actor stressed that GHD actors need to be *"comfortable with learning new skill sets"* (INFML 7). The same respondent acknowledged that although GHD actors may be unfamiliar with certain aspects of their roles, it behooves them to be curious learners while facing uncertainties and being willing to acquire the necessary knowledge and skills to build proficiency.

Countering and Managing Mis-and-Disinformation

Regarding GHD actors' ability to manage or counter mis- and disinformation, about half of Informal GHD actors vocalized the ramifications that social media, mis- and disinformation had both on pandemic response efforts and on the credibility of GHD actors and public health practitioners:

Another Informal GHD actor reflected on politicians' roles in the politicization and polarization of public health to foster their personal agendas:

Sharing a similar outlook, another Informal GHD actor opined:

6. **Communication Knowledge Gaps**

This section presents Informal GHD actors' expression of gaps in knowledge on the use of various communication formats, such as written, verbal, public speaking, elevator pitches, and crisis/risk communication, in GHD practice. Participants in this group highlighted the lack of knowledge on how to promptly access and share access information and how to communicate in emergencies to mitigate mistrust and loss of credibility.

Access to Information and Knowledge Dissemination

Looking back on GHD actors' knowledge of how to access and share information during the pandemic, about a third of Informal GHD actors underscored the need for timely access and dissemination of accurate information in emergencies. These actors

201

stated that GHD actors were either not equipped for this purpose or unwilling to share

information:

> *"Knowledge-sharing was a huge challenge early on, obviously. The failure of countries to be upfront and transparent about what was happening within their own countries with respect to the virus, and I say China particularly, but others were, too. It was really catastrophic and allowed the spread of the virus, and it still remains a challenge obviously to this day"* (INFML 5).

Another Informal GHD actor commented on the rate at which information was

disseminated to various populations based on their geographical locations. They stated

that last-mile populations or those residing in the hinterlands did not receive information

in real-time:

> *"Access to knowledge, information, and communication is important [as well as] the ability to have an adequately trained workforce to disseminate that knowledge. Most of the time, the information reached out to the urban and maybe peri-urban areas but not to the rural areas in terms of what was going on and how they should actually protect themselves. Another thing: What was the penetration of communication in the country? There might have been a sort of global knowledge dissemination, but the timeliness of that information, how swiftly it actually got to a country and from the country down to the regional and local levels, that's a big question"* (INFML 6)

Communication in Emergencies

Regarding communication in public health emergencies, a few Informal GHD

actors commented on the need for GHD actors to know how to communicate during the

pandemic to keep the public informed and encourage the uptake of preventive measures

by the community:

> *"What worked was to have clear, honest communication early on, frequent communication from those in power to the public, not to politicize the issue for political gains but to put the public wellbeing first and foremost. The delivery of the message was important to follow the science as best as we knew it at the time in terms of what needed to be implemented to prevent the spread of that virus. And then having a population that actually had trust in its government that was not used to being manipulated, that was somewhat inoculated against the disinformation being utilized to achieve political ends at the expense of great loss*

of life. So, I think having that the communication was important, having the trust in the government was important" (INFML 5).

The same respondent expressed GHD actors' inability to communicate scientific information to non-scientific or non-academic audiences in an unambiguous manner, resulting in a lack of comprehension on the listener's part:

> *"It's a big failure in global health that a lot of folks don't really capture this and understand that how we communicate in academia is so vastly different than how politicians communicate. We don't use the same language. And so, if they're speaking Swahili to a Norwegian, it's not gonna work"* (INFML 5).

Erosion of Public Trust

While reflecting on the public's mistrust of public health practitioners and policymakers, some Informal GHD actors discussed the framing of public health messaging during the pandemic, which they said often made it hard for the public to discern facts from fallacy or, depending on their political affiliation, influenced whether they accepted or rejected that information altogether:

> *"Going back to the chain of command at the Federal level, the President is ultimately in charge. The next in command is the Secretary of Health and Human Services, and the next in command is the Director of the CDC. That's the natural chain of command. Now, the Director of the CDC was Robert Redfield, and he was basically invisible. He never went before the cameras he didn't make much of any public comment, so the CDC was largely invisible. Alex Azar, who was the Secretary of HHS, was largely pushed aside by Trump. Trump did not like delegating communication. He liked to be one in the public eye more than anything else. He liked to appear in control, even though he didn't know what he was doing, and he made all sorts of outlandish claims, so that left a huge gap. And that's when Dr. Tony Fauci came in as kind of a spokesperson, if you will. And he lasted as long until Trump no longer trusted him or wanted him around either"* (INFML 3).

Research Question 4: How do Global Health Diplomacy actors define Global Health

Diplomacy in a post-COVID era?

This section presents Core, Multistakeholder, and Informal GHD actors'

definitions of Global Health Diplomacy in a post-COVID era, taking into account the

knowledge skills and core competencies they had proposed.

Core GHD Actors' Definition of Global Health Diplomacy

Core GHD actors' definitions of Global Health Diplomacy in a post-COVID era

recognized the far-reaching impact of global health challenges and the interconnection

between health and all sectors of society. A few GHD actors asserted that health is always

on the agenda, which requires that GHD actors are equipped with the necessary

knowledge, skills, and competencies to properly negotiate and advocate for the health of

the populations or countries they represent. GHD actors also acknowledged how health

could be leveraged to foster international relations amongst countries, create avenues for

cooperation and collaboration, and advance foreign policy priorities for better global

health outcomes. The definitions of Global Health Diplomacy in a post-COVID era

advanced by Core GHD actors are captured in the quote below and in Appendix 6:

> *"Global Health Diplomacy is based on the recognition that health issues
> permeate everything else, virtually everything else in life. The health of a
> population has an enormous impact on its ability to educate its children and its
> ability to have worker productivity and economic development. I think that health
> diplomacy is about recognizing how deeply these health issues influence security,
> environment, climate, economic development, education, equity for women, and
> equity for marginalized groups. To me, Global Health Diplomacy is selling that
> reality to people so that the health people do get to have a seat at the table for
> those conversations"* (CORE 7).

Multistakeholder Actors' Definition of Global Health Diplomacy

Multistakeholder GHD actors' definition of Global Health Diplomacy highlighted the need for a multifaceted, evidence-based, and scientific approach to addressing global health challenges. Respondents emphasized the importance of global multistakeholder communication, coordination, and collaboration that includes the community and local organizations in outbreak prevention and response efforts. These actors' definitions also emphasized the importance of a One Health approach that considers the intricate link between human beings and their shared ecosystem with animals and plants, as well as the impact of climate change on health. The definitions of Global Health Diplomacy in a post-COVID era by Multistakeholder GHD actors are presented below:

> *"Global Health Diplomacy is building trusted relationships and keeping science and evidence at the front, so that we do things and base our decisions and our actions on science and data, but also ensuring that we don't work in silos, that we work across our partners, across countries, across disciplines, across ministries. So that very, very collaborative openness is really essential. I think we learned that the hard way."* (MSTK 7).

Informal Actors' Definition of Global Health Diplomacy

Informal GHD actors' definitions of Global Health Diplomacy in a post-COVID era elicited a collaborative approach to increase global surveillance and preparedness for future outbreaks by strengthening countries' capacity and health systems. Actors also underscored the role of Global Health Diplomacy in improving humanity's well-being by bridging scientific discovery and implementation for improved health outcomes. This group also stated that understanding the present-day and evolving geopolitical landscape, as well as the interconnectedness between humans, animals, and plants, was critical to developing practical and effective solutions to health challenges. Informal GHD Actors' definitions of Global Health Diplomacy in a post-COVID era are outlined below:

> *"Global Health Diplomacy requires not only the recognition of the importance of human health in international affairs but also One Health, recognizing that human health is inextricably linked to healthy animals, plants, environments, and ecosystems"* (INFML 3).

A Synthesis of Global Health Diplomacy Definitions

The definitions of Global Health Diplomacy by the Core, Multistakeholder, and Informal GHD actors underscored the importance of international collaboration with GHD counterparts from other ministries, disciplines, and populations. These actors cautioned against working in silos and called for GHD actors across the world to band together to make the world safer and healthier. These actors also explained that some collaborative relationships can be technical in nature, where the GHD actors exchange technical skills and competencies to solve health problems. The Core, Multistakeholder, and Informal GHD actors also expressed the need for technical and scientific risk assessments to determine how best to address developmental needs within the population.

The Multistakeholder and Informal GHD actors' definitions of Global Health Diplomacy had some similarities around the importance of coordination for pandemic preparedness to improve health outcomes and how foreign policy objectives impact health. These definitions recognized Global Health Diplomacy as a means of bringing some level of coordination at the intersection of health and foreign policy in an otherwise messy and uncoordinated world. The actors also recognized the complexity of the world we live in that makes it impossible to achieve all of one's goals. These actors emphasized the need for coordination with the international community to ensure foreign aid and critical supplies benefit the populations or communities who need them the most.

The Informal and Multistakeholder GHD actors also acknowledged how quickly diseases can spread across international borders, which they stated requires that GHD actors work proactively to prevent the spread of diseases instead of being reactive. They further emphasized how efforts to advocate for and protect the health of the community contribute to securitizing health at the domestic and international levels. They asserted the need to equip local health facilities to ensure early detection and reporting of disease outbreaks as well as leveraging One Health, considering the link between human beings, plants, animals, and their shared environment. Both groups also noted the effect of climate change on the health of humans, their food supply, the sustainability of the environment, and the health of the planet and how health policies ultimately affect these domains.

Amongst the GHD definitions advanced by the Core and Multistakeholder actors, respondents recognized that health is intricately linked to other sectors, which they said requires that these multisectoral actors be at the table when health decisions are being made. These respondents reiterated that multisectoral engagement is critical to health security, particularly calling for the involvement of local and community stakeholders in identifying and reporting infectious disease outbreaks.

The Informal GHD actors' definitions of GHD emphasize communication with stakeholders to first understand the context in which GHD actors find themselves, in addition to collaborating and coordinating to determine the countries' health systems' capacity to identify existing gaps. They further explained the need to collaborate with other stakeholders to meet these gaps, particularly in the area of pandemic preparedness. Informal GHD actors underlined GHD actors' ability to negotiate and to understand the terms, motivations, and desired outcomes of negotiations. They also acknowledged that the role of diplomats is defined by their countries' foreign policy objectives and would be even more so in a post-COVID era, considering the ongoing shifts in the geopolitical landscapes.

The GHD definitions by Core GHD actors recognize that health is always on the agenda and intersects with all other sectors of human existence. They insisted that GHD actors must leverage their diplomatic capacities and assets to foster relationship-building amongst other countries by finding areas of convergence while limiting areas of divergence.

Finally, the Global Health Diplomacy Definition by Multistakeholder GHD actors asserted that GHD engagements and decisions are grounded in science and evidence-based practice but also partnership-driven to facilitate the exchange of ideas beyond the US to other countries.

Aim 4: Generate a summary of core competency requirements for GHD practice in a post-COVID era based on data from each GHD actor level.

In the figure below, the Researcher presents a summary of Global Health Diplomacy core competencies as expressed by Core, Multistakeholder, and Informal GHD actors in their responses to the knowledge, skills, and core competencies required for effective GHD practice in a post-COVID era. The data represented in the figure draws from GHD actors' responses to RQ1, RQ2, and RQ3 that had been distilled across the Interpersonal, Technical, Critical and Analytical Thinking, Practical, Learning, and Communication themes, each with their corresponding sub-themes. Systemic core competencies identified in RQ3, a theme that did not feature in RQ1 and RQ2, were also included in this summary as they equally have a significant bearing on effective GHD practice, specifically in pandemic/emergency preparedness and response.

Each theme and sub-themes were synthesized to their most appropriate descriptor or label. To avoid duplication, in areas where the same theme or sub-theme appeared more than once, albeit within different categories, only one label or descriptor for each theme or sub-theme was retained. For instance, if "Leadership" appeared as a sub-theme across the Core, Multistakeholder, and Informal GHD categories, it was only represented once in the figure.

A comparative analysis of GHD core competency requirements proposed by Core, Multistakeholder, and Informal GHD actors revealed similarities and differences across each group.

Amongst all three GHD actor categories, the need for Global Health Diplomacy training was mentioned, along with a variety of interpersonal skills and abilities, critical and analytical thinking, the need for training in specific technical or intricate areas, and practical or real-world GHD experience. The Core, Multistakeholder, and Informal GHD actors also mentioned GHD actors' ability to learn from the past, different formats of communication, inclusive of how to communicate during crises or emergencies, and the knowledge of stakeholders and multisectoral engagement.

Amongst the Core and Multistakeholder GHD actors, shared core competencies include collaboration and teamwork, pandemic/emergency preparedness and response, the understanding how to access timely information, and the knowledge and mastery of foreign languages.

Among the Core and Informal GHD actors, shared core competencies include understanding project management and financial resource management and utilization, understanding data analysis and statistics, mentorship and peer-learning opportunities, understanding of global health instruments, regulations, and treaties, understanding of performance frameworks and capacity assessments, the knowledge of how to conduct lockdowns and social distancing measures, and how understanding how to manage the erosion of public trust.

Among Multistakeholder and Informal GHD actors, the knowledge of computers (informatics) and web technology, leadership, negotiation, and managing misinformation and disinformation were also shared core competencies. Other core competencies that featured isolatedly within specific actor categories have been included in the summary as well.

The figure below summarizes the specific Global Health Diplomacy Core Competency areas recommended by Core, Multistakeholder, and Informal GHD actors.

Figure 5

Summary of GHD core competency requirements for GHD practice

Global Health Diplomacy Specific Competency Area						
Interpersonal competency areas	GHD actors should have knowledge of and demonstrate cross-cultural awareness and cultural sensitivity	Leadership: how to lead, and when to lead	Partnership, collaboration, and cooperation development	Personable or Soft Skills	Diplomacy and Negotiation	Transparency in partnerships, communica-tions, and leadership	
Technical competency areas	Need for training in specific technical or intricate areas, which, albeit	Expertise in Scientific, Clinical, or Technical Intricate Area	Emergency Preparedness and Response	Financial Knowledge, Stewardship, Accountability (supply chain logistics)	Global Health / Public Health	Government Culture vs. NGO Culture	Project Reporting, Monitoring, and Evaluation

	diverse, reflect the diversity in GHD requirements	Informatics, Data systems, and management	Performance frameworks and Country Capacity Assessments				
Critical and Analytical competency areas	Knowledge of how to evaluate and validate credible sources of information	Having the technical expertise to reliably assess information quality for GHD practice		Understanding One Health and systems-thinking			
GHD Practice competency areas	Need for practice and training in specific areas, which, albeit diverse, reflect the diversity in GHD requirements	Agenda and Priority-Setting	Bilateral and Multilateral Negotiations	Contextual and Situational awareness	Global Health Diplomacy Practice or Practical Experience	Global Health Security	Governmental and Non-Governmental Organizations
		International Regulations/Regulatory Processes and Governance Frameworks	Knowledge of Stakeholders and Multisectoral Engagement	Mentoring, Peer, and Cross-Cultural Exchanges	Emergency/Pandemic Preparedness and Response	Understanding of US Interagency Protocols	Public Health/Global Health/Health Policy & Economics
		Understanding politics, power dynamics, the geopolitical and GHD landscapes	Knowledge of how to counter or manage mis- and disinformation	On-the-job learning, mentorship, and peer-learning			
GHD Learning competency areas		Understanding and having the flexibility for practical on-the-job Learning	Understanding the Role of the Private Sector	Engaging in Case Studies and Real-world Simulation Exercises	Knowledge of how to counter or manage mis- and disinformation		
Communication competency areas	Effective communication is a key competency area for all GHD actors, and they need to have intensive training in multiple forms of communication.		Forms of Communication (verbal, nonverbal)	Mediums of Communication (report, Zoom, video, elevator speeches, public speaking)	Types of communication (Risk, technical, crisis with transparency and honesty)	Knowledge and mastery of foreign languages	

This chapter presented GHD actors' responses to the required knowledge, skills, and competencies for GHD. The study findings will be discussed in the next chapter.

Chapter Five: Discussion

This study set out to achieve four aims, which were to identify the skills and core competencies that Core, Multistakeholder, and Informal GHD actors need to practice GHD in a post-COVID era, identify the technical knowledge gaps that exist within each set of GHD actors, present GHD actors definitions of Global Health Diplomacy, and lastly, propose a summary of GHD actors core competencies for a post-COVID era. The study utilized a Grounded Theory, descriptive qualitative design to capture GHD actors' viewpoints, trends, beliefs, or perceptions on knowledge, skills, or core competencies to inform or affect GHD practice in a post-COVID era (Glaser & Strauss, 2017).

The interview questions were posed in an open-ended format to allow for an in-depth exploration of participants' responses to the research questions. Participants responded to the questions based on what they considered to be the most essential skills, core competencies, and technical knowledge gaps based on their experiences. Questions were not shared with the interviewees ahead of time. Therefore, the responses provided were non-rehearsed and from their own perspectives. This explanation may account for areas of overlap or similarities in participants' responses across all Research Questions. Alternatively, respondents may have wanted to avoid being repetitive in their response if they felt a particular skill could also be a core competency and would have chosen not to mention it a second time.

Aim 1: Required Skills and Competencies for GHD Practice in a Post-COVID Era

RQ1: What skills do GHD actors need for effective Global Health Diplomacy practice in a post-COVID era?

Interpersonal Skills

Interpersonal, relational, or soft skills were a salient theme across all the GHD actor categories, which is unsurprising considering Global Health Diplomacy is based on personal interactions and relationships. Personal attributes such as empathy, active listening, humility, patience, flexibility, emotional intelligence, cross-cultural awareness, and cultural sensitivity were underscored as necessary for engaging with others, starting from those on one's team (Pancheshnikov et al., 2023). Amongst the Core GHD actors, being genuinely interested in learning about people and other cultures was vital for negotiations and in-person interactions. Core GHD actors often interact with other Global Health Diplomacy Actors from different countries, such as Health Attaches, Ministers of Foreign Affairs, Ambassadors, and Ministers of Health, which requires them to be adept at relationship-building and finding areas of convergence within foreign policy priorities. For the Multistakeholder GHD actors, the ability to see others' perspectives, understand their counterpart's positionality and the context in which discussions or negotiations were taking place, and be open-minded helped foster trust, mutual understanding, collaboration, and cooperation (Abdi, Lega & Ravagi, 2021). The World Health Organization, the World Health Assembly, and the United Nations are examples of multilateral fora within which negotiations for health occur. For example, ongoing negotiations for the amendment of the International Health Regulations and the ratification of the Pandemic Agreement require the aforementioned personal attributes for consensus-building, collaboration, and cooperation amongst multilateral Global Health Diplomacy actors. The Informal GHD actors highlighted the ability to self-reflect and understand political, institutional, and organizational cultures as 'really important' for

GHD practice. For example, this group of actors includes representatives of international non-governmental organizations who may be implementing programs or intervening in a host country with cultural norms and practices that may differ from their home countries. Therefore, such GHD actors would need to understand the host country's sociopolitical, economic, and environmental landscape and its governance and regulatory processes and how this may affect the scope of the international NGO's operations in the country.

Technical Skills

The findings show significant diversity in the technical skills required by each group of GHD actors, which may reflect the diversity in the different forms of Global Health Diplomacy. For example, emergency response, research, peacebuilding, or medical exchanges can reflect multiplicity in the roles and responsibilities of GHD actors. The Core and Informal GHD categories mentioned the importance of project management, the ability to manage and utilize financial resources appropriately, as well as GHD actors' ability to analyze data and understand statistical or epidemiological trends (Jahn et al., 2022). Project management and financial stewardship abilities may reflect the need for accountability to the US Legislative branch that regulates spending policies, considering the United States is the most significant funder of global health efforts worldwide and the highest donor of foreign assistance.

Among the Core GHD actors, respondents underlined the importance of having a clinical or public health background (Van den Broucke, 2020) to be a Global Health Diplomat. The emphasis on this ability may reflect the challenges experienced by non-health GHD actors to respond to the demands of the COVID-19 pandemic, which require an understanding of critical areas such as epidemiology and disease transmission, as well as performing the key public health functions that are disease prevention, health protection, and health promotion.

Conversely, other Core GHD actors asserted that diplomatic interactions benefitted more from actors being generalists and having personality skills, considering they could rely on other technical experts and personal experience or develop the required skills when necessary. This outlook could be due to the sheer number of issues and topics that Core GHD actors must deal with whilst stationed abroad for which they may not have been trained. Within the Core GHD participants, GHD actors' ability to understand the functioning of logistics and supply chain systems and the epidemiology of disease transmission was also articulated, as well as having technical expertise that spanned several domains.

Within the Multistakeholder GHD actors, there was a stronger emphasis on the need for a clinical or public/global health background and expertise in a 'specific technical or intricate area,' which was also wide-ranging, as previously explained. Many of the suggested technical skills were science-related, clinical, or biomedical. These skills appeared to reflect specific needs elicited by the recent pandemic and past outbreaks, such as epidemiology, developing medical countermeasures, and drug or vaccine trials. For Multistakeholder GHD actors, being an expert was also accentuated as a means for establishing trust and credibility amongst one's peers and counterparts, which created the path for diplomacy.

The Multistakeholder GHD actors' mention of the need for credibility may also stem from the erosion of public trust that public health officials and health organizations like WHO experienced during the pandemic due to conflicting public health messaging and the politicization of public health. Amongst this group, other domains, such as the need for actors to understand research and the implications of sharing data, knowledge, and resources, especially during emergencies, were critical, as were key lessons learned from the recent pandemic and previous infectious disease outbreaks or epidemics.

Furthermore, being able to negotiate health or scientific technicalities such as drug trials and the rapid development, production, and distribution of vaccines during the pandemic was deemed important, particularly whilst dealing with a novel virus. Multistakeholder GHD actors' assertion of the need for accountability in financial resource management and having the flexibility to preposition or reallocate limited resources in emergencies may indicate the need to rapidly deploy resources at short notice, bypassing the sometimes lengthy and multilayered financial approval processes.

The Informal GHD actors reiterated the importance of GHD actors familiarizing themselves with the One Health concept (CDC.gov, 2023) and other systems-thinking approaches that lent themselves well to emergency responses and ethical considerations for public health interventions (Czabanowska & Kuhlmann, 2021), especially at the population level. The need for systems thinking may stem from the acknowledgment of the intersection between health and other sectors, the impact of COVID-19 on all sectors, particularly on trade and travel, and the short and long-term effects on global economies, which are yet to be fully understood.

Critical and Analytical Thinking Skills

Core, Multistakeholder, and Informal GHD actors articulated the importance of using logic and objectivity in decision-making, which relied on the actors' ability to evaluate and synthesize information. It is common for GHD actors to make decisions without having all the facts or all the data necessary. Often, GHD actors rely on just-in-time information, which underscores the need for them to be able to access credible and timely information and might explain why this sub-theme featured across all three GHD actor groups.

Within the Core GHD actor group, this process required the ability to balance risk and uncertainty by assessing potential outcomes and unintended consequences of one's decisions, and considering the implications on bilateral and multilateral relationships. For the Multistakeholder GHD actors, the post-COVID era warrants an appraisal of how the GHD landscape is evolving and how changes to political, socioeconomic, environmental, and legal contexts may influence future global health partnerships and drivers of equity or inequity (Khullar & Chokshi, 2018; Abdi, Lega, & Ravagi, 2021).

As demonstrated by a review of the literature on the history and evolution of GHD in the second chapter, Global Health Diplomacy has been defined by global health events that have directly impacted multiple sectors across countries and health negotiations. These changes may account for why the Multistakeholder GHD actors underscored the need for GHD actors' ability to understand the situational contexts and their broader effects on the population.

For Informal GHD actors, an understanding of local, regional, and international contexts and countries' capacity to prevent, detect, and respond to disease outbreaks was indispensable for GHD practice. The need for this skill may reflect specific levels of intervention or program implementation by Informal GHD actors. For example, implementing emergency or development programs effectively would require multilevel, multisectoral coordination, communication, and collaboration to identify and address existing capacity and response gaps.

Practical or Practice-Based Skills

Across this theme, GHD actors' responses showed similarities concerning practicing Global Health Diplomacy. The need for Global Health Diplomacy training was mentioned across the Core, Multistakeholder, and Informal GHD actor categories (Voss et al., 2021). Some definitions of Global Health Diplomacy describe the field as 'emerging,' which may explain the need for GHD training. Conversely, this need may have also been elicited by how much this field has and continues to change in scope of practice and the growing number of GHD actors.

Core and Multistakeholder GHD actors emphasized the need for practical or real-world GHD experience as essential for Global Health Diplomacy actors. Having real-world experience was integral to initiating and navigating bilateral, multilateral, national, or local engagements (Boujnah, 2022), which supported a better understanding of the populations GHD actors represented and the context in which these interactions occurred (Asadi-Lari et al., 2021). In addition, real-life experience can also confer a practical understanding of actual events and how to navigate the demands and challenges thereof that are lacking in theoretical scenarios.

For Multistakeholder and Informal actors, negotiation skills were crucial for GHD practice, as was the need for GHD actors to be adaptable, flexible, and amenable to taking risks, particularly in emergencies (Reina Ortiz et al., 2021) and when dealing with multisectoral stakeholders and host governments.

Core GHD actors noted how health intersects with other sectors and US foreign policy objectives. Thus, GHD actors must understand how to adequately represent US interests and priorities, which is central to their role (Fidler, 2011). Multistakeholder GHD actors upheld the need for leadership abilities and GHD actors' understanding of the role of public health in health promotion (Levin-Zahmir et al., 2021) and health protection. Furthermore, they recommended the infusion of human and financial resources to support these functions and strengthen public health systems, making them more resilient to global shocks and better prepared for the growing burden of non-communicable and infectious diseases.

Informal GHD actors discussed how knowledge and engagement of stakeholders helped facilitate partnership development. Global Health Diplomacy actors must work with a wide variety of multidisciplinary stakeholders from the public and private sectors who may need to be consulted and informed or whose approval may need to be obtained prior to engaging with the host country or communities. These actors also stressed that emergency preparedness and response skills are critical for GHD practice, which may reflect personal real-life practice gaps based on lived experiences or their observation of gaps in other GHD actors' abilities that the COVID-19 pandemic response spotlighted.

Unlike the Core and Multistakeholder GHD categories, Informal GHD actors emphasized the need to understand the evolving Global Health Diplomacy landscape and US foreign policy priorities through a geopolitical lens, as well as the interplay of political will and power on current and future GHD objectives (Vuković, 2020). The COVID-19 pandemic ushered in a period where health rose to the top of foreign policy agendas, becoming a significant foreign policy priority. However, competing economic and sociopolitical priorities can make it challenging to garner sustained interest from policymakers and decision-makers. A transition in leadership can also affect whether certain priorities are maintained or shelved amidst the turnover in administrative leadership or the desire of incumbents to distinguish themselves from their predecessors.

Furthermore, ongoing geopolitical rivalry and tensions, such as between the United States, Russia, and China, can have far-reaching effects as countries grapple with the repercussions of the pandemic on global and domestic economies. Informal GHD actors also raised concerns about the implications of public health ethics in emergencies and the 'blanket' application of biomedical ethical considerations, which are better suited for individuals than population health interventions. These concerns may also be a reflection of the stark inequities in the lack of COVID-19 vaccine availability, accessibility, and affordability and the disparities in healthcare access witnessed within the United States and in other LMICs over the past years that preexisted COVID-19.

Additionally, the juxtaposition of COVID-19 preventive, non-pharmaceutical countermeasures, such as masking and social distancing measures against public health ethical principles, beyond just beneficence, respect for autonomy, non-maleficence, and distributive justice, is critical. Thus, Informal GHD actors underlined the importance of GHD actors' ability to understand public health ethics and their systematic application in public health interventions to "clarify, prioritize and justify possible courses of public health action based on ethical principles, values and beliefs of stakeholders, and scientific and other information" (CDC, 2022).

Learning Skills

The need for GHD actors to learn how to access and utilize credible information in a timely manner, especially in health emergencies, was underscored by Core and

Multistakeholder GHD actors (Luh & Baltag, 2021). Emergency responses are often fast-paced and require the rapid deployment and positioning of essential resources and teams to respond to a crisis. They also necessitate real-time information sharing to facilitate adequate coordination and proper utilization of resources. Core GHD actors insisted on the importance of learning how to maintain formal and reliable informal communication channels and GHD actors' ability to make sound decisions amid uncertainty and emerging or changing information (CFR, 2017). Considering the unprecedented rejection, polarization, and discrediting of public health during the COVID pandemic, Multistakeholder and Informal GHD actors felt strongly that GHD actors must learn how to manage and counter mis- and disinformation (Vériter, Bjola, & Koops, 2020).

Communication Skills

All three categories of GHD actors recognized the importance of communication in all its different formats: written, spoken, presentations, and non-verbal. Communication underpins interpersonal interactions, relationship-building, negotiations, mediation, and advocacy, which are central to Global Health Diplomacy and may explain why this was a common theme across all respondent categories. The importance of clarity, conciseness, and the ability to address non-scientific or non-technical audiences was also mentioned as inherent to effective communication by Core, Multistakeholder, and Informal GHD actors (Zemmel et al., 2021). By and large, among Core and Multistakeholder GHD groups, the GHD actors' knowledge of foreign languages (Lazzarini, 2015) was deemed essential in cross-cultural interactions, negotiations, and communication (Biletska, Lastovskyi, & Semchynskyy, 2023). Languages can be a gateway into host country cultures. They may facilitate direct interactions and a more nuanced understanding of what is being discussed, which may sometimes not be captured by direct translation or interpretation.

Core GHD actors' ability to 'read the room' and accurately understand the often-imperceptible forms of communication, such as a person's body language, hearing what was not being said, and being able to ask big-picture questions, was essential for diplomatic interactions. The Core GHD actor group also mentioned the ability to communicate risk as a critical GHD skill, as well as the ability of GHD actors to assess how social media influences population behavior, specifically with regard to the uptake of or rejection of public health recommendations. The prevalence of mis- and disinformation on social media platforms was rife during the pandemic and played a significant role in public perception of scientific and non-scientific discourse and efforts to contain the spread of the virus. The effect of this unprecedented infodemic is worth exploring for a better understanding of population-level effects in a post-COVID era.

For Multistakeholder GHD actors, an understanding of the context, purpose of communication, and the designated audience was primordial, particularly in negotiations. For example, public health messaging should ideally be curated for specific audiences based on the listener's unique characteristics to facilitate understanding, agency, and adaptation of communication style, formats, and tone. For Informal GHD actors, GHD actors' communication during emergency responses and the ability to distill their message to a diverse group of stakeholders supports the dissemination of information and facilitates multisectoral coordination and collaboration (Kickbusch & Liu, 2022). It could also help provide clarity on stakeholders' roles and responsibilities, allowing for a more harmonious emergency response.

The table below presents an analysis of responses for required skills for GHD practice based on Core, Multistakeholder, and Informal GHD actors' responses. Areas, where a central theme was not mentioned in the GHD actors' responses are left blank. The 'x' represents the GHD actors' responses corresponding to a specific sub-theme.

For example, all three GHD actor categories highlighted the importance of having various interpersonal or soft skills, the ability to synthesize, analyze, and evaluate information, the need for GHD training, and a mastery of different communication styles and formats using other mediums. The Core and Informal GHD actors mentioned understanding project management, data analysis and statistics, and financial resource stewardship. The Core and Multistakeholder actors underscored the importance of knowing how to access information in a timely manner, having practical Global Health Diplomacy experience, and knowledge and mastery of foreign languages. The Multistakeholder and Informal GHD actors shared similarities in the need for GHD actors to be flexible, adaptable, calculated risk-takers, and know how to negotiate, manage, or counteract misinformation and disinformation.

Conversely, some skills did appear only within one GHD actor category. For example, understanding of logistics and supply chain management for Core GHD actors, having research and computer skills for the Multistakeholder GHD actors or understanding One Health for Informal GHD actors. However, this may not necessarily imply that these skills are only relevant to actors within the groups in which they were identified. The role of GHD actors can be very diverse, changing, and evolving as needed. Thus, the skills below reflect GHD actors' roles and responsibilities during the COVID-19 pandemic and those recommended for GHD practice, now and in the future, based on the function GHD actors may be required to perform. Arguably, the more

diverse the skillsets that GHD actors possess, the better equipped they will be to practice

GHD in a post-COVID era.

Table 18

Data Analysis Table of Required Skills for Core, Multistakeholder, and Informal GHD Actors

RQ 1: Skills				
Theme	Sub-theme	CORE	MSTK	INFML
Interpersonal	Mix of interpersonal skills	x	x	x
	Project Management	x		x
	Logistics and Supply Chain	x		
	Financial Resource Management and Utilization	x		x
	Data Analysis and Statistics	x		x
	Epidemiology and Disease Transmission	x		
	Health or Scientific Expertise	x		
	Broad Mix of Technical Expertise	x		
	Non-Health/ Non-Scientific Expertise	x		
	Generalist	x		
Technical	Research		x	
	Computer Skills		x	
	Technical Negotiations		x	
	Public Health or Global Health Expertise		x	
	Understanding Implications for Data, Knowledge, and Resource Sharing		x	
	Technical Expertise or Background		x	
	Flexibility in Resource Allocation and Utilization		x	
	Financial Management and Accountability		x	
	One Health and Understanding of Systems Thinking			x

	Clinical Expertise or Healthcare Background			x
Critical and Analytical Thinking	Ability to synthesize, analyze, and evaluate information objectively and logically to make informed and sound decisions	x	x	x
Practical or Practice-Based	Practical or Real-World Global Health Diplomacy Experience	x	x	
	Multisectorality in Diplomacy	x		
	Understanding the Intersection between Health and Foreign Policy	x		
	Global Health Diplomacy Training	x	x	x
	Individual and Institutional Adaptability, Flexibility, and Risk-Taking		x	x
	Negotiation Skills		x	x
	Leadership Skills		x	
	Understanding the Role of Public Health		x	
	Knowledge of Stakeholders and Multisectoral Engagement			x
	Pandemic/Emergency Preparedness and Response			x
	Understanding US Foreign Policy Works and its Impact on Global Health			x
	Understanding the GHD Landscape			x
	Understanding Political and Power Dynamics			x
	Understanding Public Health Ethics and Ethical Implications			x
Learning	Access to Timely Information	x	x	
	Informed Decision-making Using New or Emerging Data	x		
	Managing Misinformation and Disinformation		x	x
Communication	Communication types and formats	Communication [Written, verbal, elevator pitches, PowerPoint, Synthesizing information, Public Speaking, Risk communication, media relations, persuasiveness	Communication [Written, verbal, elevator pitches, PowerPoint, Synthesizing information, Public Speaking, Risk communication]	Communication [Written, verbal, elevator pitches, PowerPoint, Synthesizing information, Public Speaking, Risk communication]

	x	x
Knowledge and Mastery of Foreign Languages		
The role of the Media and social media on Population Behavior	x	

RQ2: What Core Competencies do GHD actors need for effective Global Health Diplomacy practice in a post-COVID era?

Interpersonal Competencies

When discussing interpersonal competencies for GHD practice, Multistakeholder GHD actors highlighted cross-cultural awareness and cultural sensitivity as foundational competencies for building relationships (Pancheshnikov et al., 2023). These competencies can also facilitate an understanding or appreciation for the GHD actors' counterparts' preferences, attitudes, or behaviors that may affect receptivity or acceptability during interpersonal interactions. Among the Multistakeholder and Informal GHD categories, similarities in interpersonal core competencies, such as leadership and transparency, in association with other personal attributes like active listening, empathy, honesty, trustworthiness, servant leadership, and legitimacy or personal credibility, were noted. The need for these competencies may have been underscored by the challenges in crisis leadership that public leaders faced domestically and on the global stage during the pandemic. Some of these issues resulted in the politicization, polarization, and loss of credibility and trust in public and scientific leadership figures. Multistakeholder GHD respondents also underscored the ability of GHD actors to develop key partnerships. Strategic partnership development can bring together the knowledge and resources from actors across the public and private sectors to jointly address complex global challenges like COVID-19. The Core GHD actors did not share any interpersonal competencies specific to this theme. A possible explanation for this could be that this group had already shared an elaborate list of interpersonal abilities whilst responding to the question about the skills required for GHD practice. Whilst these interpersonal skills may also apply to core competencies, they may not have shared them in their responses to this question in particular to avoid being repetitive.

Technical Competencies

The technical competencies advanced by Core and Multistakeholder GHD actors within this theme were quite distinct from each other, which are most likely reflective of the diversity in the roles of interviewees. Core GHD actors highlighted specific technical competency domains, including financial knowledge and stewardship, navigating the challenges of complicated logistics and supply chains, and understanding the difference in institutional cultures between government entities and non-governmental organizations. The Core GHD actors also underscored the need for technical expertise or understanding 'how science works' (Rungius & Flink, 2020) as pertains to the demands of preparing and responding to outbreaks. The ability to understand scientific data and communicate it clearly and concisely to policy and decision-makers to galvanize action toward a desired outcome is critical in the practice of GHD. These actors mentioned specific competency areas, including epidemiology, disease surveillance, and diagnostics testing, which mirror the priority areas within the COVID-19 response, and require knowledge and expertise that most generalists may not have, even if they may be skilled communicators.

Similarly, several Multistakeholder GHD actor technical competencies centered around emergency preparedness and response efforts, including GHD actors' ability to manage data systems and monitor and evaluate projects. The ability to generate end-of-project reports was also emphasized, as this responsibility, though vital, is sometimes overlooked at the height of emergency responses. Multistakeholder GHD actors also asserted the need for GHD actors to have scientific, public/global health, or clinical expertise, which can support their understanding and implementation of core public health functions in emergency and non-emergency scenarios that require health protection and health promotion policies and interventions. Informal GHD actors did not share any technical competencies pertaining to this theme. However, they did share a variety of specific practice-based skills and practice-based competencies below, which may reflect their need for the demonstrable ability for GHD actors to perform specific tasks within and outside the scope of their roles and responsibilities when needed.

Critical and Analytical Thinking Competencies

The critical and analytical thinking competencies for Core GHD actors were identical to those mentioned within the Skills domain regarding GHD actors' abilities to find, assess, and use information for sound decision-making. However, this theme was not reflected in the Multistakeholder and Informal GHD actors' responses to GHD actors' essential core competencies. As previously explained, the interviewer asked open-ended questions that participants may have responded to with any answers of their choosing. Thus, the absence of this theme is less likely to be an indicator of importance or lack thereof; instead, the likelihood that a particular response may not have been at the forefront of respondents' minds at the time the question was asked.

Practical or Practice-Based Competencies

Global Health Diplomacy actors' responses to required practice-based competencies and suggestions for training domains to enhance GHD practice were remarkably diverse, considering the diversity of participants interviewed, and their roles. When discussing other practice-based competencies apart from training, Core GHD actors' recommendations for GHD practice-based competencies included traditional diplomatic and negotiation skills and abilities, foreign policy priority-setting, and bilateral and multilateral engagement (Tago, 2017). These specific areas are very much ingrained into the daily functions of Core GHD actors or Global Health Diplomats. Respondents in this actor category also discussed the need for a skillset in cooperation and collaboration (Nkengasong, 2023) and the understanding of governance regulatory frameworks such as the International Health Regulations.

Understanding US interagency coordination was also mentioned, which can be particularly useful when initiating a whole-of-government approach for emergency response or conducting stakeholder analyses (CDC Office of Policy, Performance, and Evaluation, 2022). Stakeholder analyses can help garner information on the characteristics of key interest parties, their role in the decision-making process, their vested interests, how these stakeholders interact with each other, and the context in which these interactions occur.

Core GHD actors also highlighted the importance for GHD actors to understand how GHD is practiced in the real world, specifically highlighting the non-linear path that sometimes leads to GHD actors becoming Global Health Diplomats. For example, the US Foreign Service has five main career tracks: Consular, Political, Economic, Public Diplomacy, and Management. These Foreign Service Officers, depending on the circumstances, will be required to perform the functions of a Global Health Diplomat despite not having training in global health, public health, or a clinical background.

While discussing non-training related practical GHD competencies, Multistakeholder GHD actors emphasized the need for GHD actors' understanding and awareness of the contexts and situations in which GHD interactions were being executed, particularly in relationships with a perceived or actual power imbalance. For example, GHD actors from countries that receive foreign assistance may feel they do not have the agency to negotiate or push back against donor demands or requests they may disagree with if they perceive it may affect funding streams or future disbursements.

Across the Core, Multistakeholder, and Informal GHD actors, GHD actors' knowledge and engagement of key stakeholders was essential. Stakeholder engagement is critical in policy and program development, especially in public health interventions. The goal of this process is to ensure that proposed policies or interventions are relevant and appropriate for the people or communities for whom they are designed and to ensure adequate consideration of the end-users priorities and preferences. It can also help GHD actors understand others' interests and allow them to identify areas or avenues for cooperation, collaboration, or improvement.

Multistakeholder and Informal GHD actors also underlined real-world or practical GHD experience as an important competency. Practical experience can expose GHD actors to real-world problems or challenges in an uncontrolled environment that requires pragmatism to assess these scenarios and correctly apply specific knowledge, skills, and abilities to propose or develop suitable solutions.

Specific GHD training domains advanced by Core GHD actors included the understanding of International Regulations and other global governance frameworks

(Moore, 2022). Other areas comprised negotiating in bilateral and multilateral settings (Chattu, Pooransingh & Allahverdipour, 2021), diplomacy, mentorship, peer learning, and using case studies or simulation exercises. Training domains proposed by Multistakeholders included global health security, public health and health policy, mentorship and cross-cultural exchanges, and interpersonal competency training. The need for pandemic or emergency preparedness and response training was highlighted amongst the Core and Multistakeholder GHD respondents.

The Informal GHD actors proposed the most significant list of training domains, which may reflect the significant diversity in this actor category as reflected in the Global Health Diplomacy pyramid. They recommended that graduate and medical programs update their training curriculum to include One Health and more recent scientific discoveries (Vankova, 2022) to better equip them for modern-day health security challenges. Other training domains mentioned by Informal GHD actors included the functioning of political, governmental, and non-governmental organizations, understanding of Essential Public Health Functions, and country capacities and contexts, which are critical for these actors' success.

Informal GHD actors also affirmed the need for interdisciplinary education, training, and accreditation of the public health workforce and the integration of Essential Public Health functions into undergraduate and advanced Public Health training to strengthen health system resilience. Furthermore, the Informal GHD actors also recommended that GHD actors be trained in program management, public or global health, and health economics, as well as industrial psychology of Global Health Diplomacy. Understanding industrial psychology would require that GHD actors explore the underlying factors that influence the mind and behavior of GHD actors and how these affect the decisions they make, communications, negotiations, and interactions with each other.

Learning Competencies

The ability to learn on the job was underlined as vital for both Core and Multistakeholder GHD actors, considering the myriad of topics and competing priorities they often face (Michaud & Kates, 2013). Experiential learning can allow GHD actors to pick up new skills by observing processes and procedures and putting these into practice, preferably with initial supervision or through practice in a mentored environment. Core GHD actors pointed out the importance of understanding how the private sector operates and how GHD actors can leverage private entities' capabilities in emergencies. For example, during the COVID-19 pandemic, the private sector played a central role in vaccine development, production of personal protective equipment, and therapeutics. Core GHD actors also recommended that GHD actors adopt a learning disposition and be prepared to face questions they may not have anticipated or for which they do not have answers.

Conversely, Multistakeholder GHD actors reiterated the importance of capitalizing on policies, lessons, and recommendations from previous disease outbreaks, noting that no one was an expert on COVID-19 prior to the pandemic (Kuhlmann, Dussault, & Correia, 2021). Over the years, the response to infectious disease outbreaks and epidemics has followed a cycle of panic and neglect. This phase is typically characterized by a marked surge in funding and resources in the face of a serious health threat, followed by a chronic funding deficiency toward preparedness for future outbreaks once the news headline moves on (World Bank Group, 2017).

Informal GHD actors did not share any learning competencies within the scope of this theme. However, while discussing required skills in RQ1, half of Informal GHD actors asserted the need for actors to learn how to manage misinformation and disinformation. They also noted they had been unprepared for the massive amounts of mis- and disinformation and the politicization and polarization of public health. The Informal GHD actors may have wanted to avoid being repetitive after elaborating on these aspects in their responses to the previous question, which may explain why they were not mentioned in the required core competency section.

Communication Competencies

Communication competencies advanced by Core, Multistakeholder, and Informal GHD actors were similar to those mentioned in the Skills domain. These included proficiency in the different communication formats: written, spoken, presentations, and non-verbal, and the ability to synthesize information. The similitudes in communication skills and core competencies suggest that, in real-world practice, GHD actors may not distinguish between skills and core competencies. In addition, Core GHD actors underscored the need for GHD actors to master the art of public speaking, persuasion, and delivering an elevator pitch (Nye, 2017). These communication competencies were widely echoed by all the interviewees in this category, which may indicate their pertinence to GHD practice, particularly in their roles of representing US Foreign policy interests internationally.

In contrast, Multistakeholder GHD actors whose interactions span across multilateral fora and international stakeholders underscored GHD actors' ability to speak a foreign language, which could serve as a gateway into other cultures (Council of American Ambassadors, n.d.). Among the Informal GHD actors, being competent in communication facilitated leadership, negotiations, and diplomacy, taking into account the wide range of stakeholders they interact with to facilitate partnership development and multisectoral cooperation, coordination, or consensus building. These actors also stated that being proficient at communicating risk was essential to mitigating fear and uncertainty. These competencies are crucial when designing or implementing individual or community-based interventions or dealing with the detection, containment, and management of emergencies in the community, as was the case with previous outbreaks like Ebola.

The table below presents an analysis of responses for required core competencies for GHD practice based on Core, Multistakeholder, and Informal GHD actors' responses. Areas where a main theme was not mentioned in the GHD actors' responses are left blank. The 'x' represents the GHD actors' responses corresponding to a specific sub-theme.

Similar to Table 19, the core competencies below reflect the diversity of the roles, functions, and responsibilities of GHD actors during the COVID-19 pandemic and in the future. A few areas of similarities across all three GHD actor groups include the need for GHD actors' knowledge and engagement of stakeholders across diverse sectors and proficiency in all communication formats and mediums. Amongst the Core and Multistakeholder GHD actors, the need for GHD actors to be competent in pandemic preparedness and response was emphasized. Amongst Core and Informal GHD actors, the need for mentorship and peer learning was mentioned, while Multistakeholder and Informal GHD actors mentioned leadership and transparency as critical GHD interpersonal competencies.

However, some core competencies were mentioned specifically amongst some GHD actor groups but not in others. For example, an understanding of the host government, NGO, or institutional culture for Core GHD actors, an understanding of global health or public health for Multistakeholder GHD actors, or an understanding of country capacities or contexts for Informal GHD actors. Whilst these competencies may not have been mentioned by other GHD actors in their response to these questions, I would argue that they are relevant to all GHD actors' categories, particularly in light of global health security threats and geopolitics and how these issues would affect or change the GHD landscape.

Table 19

Data Analysis Table of Required Core Competencies for Core, Multistakeholder, and Informal GHD Actors

RQ2: Core Competencies				
Theme	Sub-theme	CORE	MSTK	INFML
	Mix of interpersonal skills	None		
Interpersonal	Cross-cultural Awareness and Cultural Sensitivity		x	
	Personable or Soft Skills		x	
	Transparency		x	x
	Leadership		x	x
	Partnership Development		x	
Technical	Financial Knowledge, Stewardship & Accountability	x		
	Technical Expertise or Technical Background	x		
	Logistics and Supply Chain	x		
	Government Culture vs NGO Culture	x		
	Project Reporting, Monitoring, and Evaluation		x	

Category	Item	Knowing how to find/assess credible information		
	Data Systems and Management		X	
	Expertise in Scientific, Clinical or Technical Intricate Area		X	
	Emergency Preparedness and Response		X	
	Global Health / Public Health		X	
Critical and Analytical Thinking				
	Diplomacy	X		
	Agenda and Priority-setting	X		
	Collaboration and Cooperation	X		
	GHD training:	X		
	International Regulations/ Regulatory Processes and Governance Frameworks	X		
	Diplomacy/Diplomatic Interactions	X		
	Pandemic/Emergency Preparedness / Response	X	X	
	Case Studies and Real-world Simulation Exercises	X		
	Bilateral and Multilateral Negotiations	X		
	Mentorship and Peer-Learning	X		X
	Understanding Global Health Diplomacy in Practice	X		
Practical or Practice-Based	Knowledge of Stakeholders and Multisectoral Engagement	X	X	X
	Negotiation	X		
	Understanding Global Governance Frameworks and Multilateral Organizations	X		
	Understanding of US Interagency Protocols	X		
	contextual and situational awareness		X	
	GHD training		X	
	Global Health Security		X	
	Public Health and Health Policy		X	
	Mentoring and Cross-Cultural Exchanges		X	
	Interpersonal Training		X	
	Global Health Diplomacy Practice or Practical Experience		X	X
	Training			X
	Functioning of Political Systems			X
	Governmental and Non-Governmental Organizations			X
	Communication			X
	Industrial Psychology			X

	Project Management			x
	Public Health/ Global Health/ Health Economics			x
	Interdisciplinary Education			x
	Country Capacities and Context			x
	Essential Public Health Functions			x
	Integration of Essential Public Health Functions into Public Health Training			x
	Public Health Workforce Training and Accreditation			x
	One Health and Recent Scientific Breakthroughs			x
Learning			On-the-job learning	
			Foreign language skills	
Communication		Communication [Written, verbal, elevator pitches, PowerPoint, Synthesizing information, Public Speaking, Risk communication, media relations, persuasiveness]	Communication for building rapport or relationships concise/ accurate communication amid limited information	Communication [Written, verbal, elevator pitches, PowerPoint, Synthesizing information, Public Speaking, Risk communication]

Aim 2: Identify Technical Knowledge Gaps for each Global Health Diplomacy Actor Category

Systemic Gaps

While discussing systemic gaps, Core, Multistakeholder, and Informal GHD actors recognized inadequate or underfunded public health infrastructure (Zapata, Buchnan & Azzopardi-Muscat, 2021; Burau et al., 2022; Biddle, Wahedi, & Bozorgmehr, 2020; Bourgeault et al., 2020). Core GHD actors called out the inequity within the US health system that often made accessibility and affordability of quality healthcare impossible for people of lower socioeconomic status (Weiner, 2020; Davison et al., 2021). They also explained how the lack of strategically positioned Foreign Service Officers in some host countries during the COVID pandemic restricted US face-to-face diplomatic interactions. This challenge resulted in the loss of formal communication channels, limited access to crucial information, and supply chain shortages (Boro & Stoll, 2022). Multistakeholder GHD actors also pointed out the lack of public health infrastructure, modern technology, and a skilled/trained public health workforce (Payne, 2021), which countries must speedily address as part of pandemic preparedness efforts. Informal GHD actors also noted the lack of infrastructure or the use of dated technology at local public health departments and globally (Zemmel et al., 2021).

Travel restrictions and stay-at-home orders during the pandemic resulted in an increased use of the internet, computers, and web technology for personal, educational, and professional use for those for whom these resources were available. For example, Zoom, Microsoft Teams, and Webex became some of the go-to communication platforms for maintaining personal and professional engagements and knowledge and information sharing amongst GHD actors and the public. However, not everyone had access to these resources or knew how to use them, which may explain why Informal GHD actors accentuated these gaps.

Multistakeholder and Informal GHD actors' responses highlighted significant gaps in countries' pandemic preparedness, detection, and response capacity before and during the pandemic. While discussing these gaps, Multistakeholder GHD actors reiterated the need to strengthen countries' surveillance, diagnostics, and response capacities, noting the challenges amid competing post-pandemic priorities (Michaud & Kates, 2013). Multistakeholder GHD actors also asserted significant gaps in essential resources such as diagnostic tests and personal protective equipment. Informal GHD actors criticized countries' failure to prioritize pandemic prevention detection and response gaps by strengthening global and domestic health infrastructure when they had the chance (Alilio et al., 2022) through the Global Health Security Agenda's efforts.

Core and Multistakeholder GHD actor groups mentioned human resource and staffing gaps: Core GHD actors also decried the lack of US embassy staff expressly trained in public health to handle health-related responsibilities, as well as insufficient research and publication on GHD actors' core competencies (Brown et al., 2018). As evidenced by the research gap identified by the literature review, only a few studies have been carried out on required GHD skills or core competencies. This gap reveals that GHD actors' knowledge, skills, and competencies have been largely unexplored due to minimal research and publications in this area. Similarly, Multistakeholder GHD actors articulated challenges in finding staff with specific skills at the height of the pandemic, insisting on the need to cross-train staff speedily and effectively. The global pandemic response was multifaceted and required tremendous human and material resources, which were in short supply, especially whilst working around the clock to mitigate the virus' spread and increase testing, treatment, and immunization.

While discussing data and essential resource gaps, Informal GHD actors emphasized the glaring inequities, such as disparities in the availability of essential resources such as PPE and diagnostic tests, particularly between more industrialized nations and LMICs. This group also pointed out COVID-19 vaccine inequity (Ledford, 2022) from vaccine hoarding (Riaz et al., 2021) or the monopoly of vaccine intellectual property rights that forestalled COVID-19 vaccine patent and technology sharing. These inequities made the vaccines inaccessible and unaffordable, especially for countries that were unable to manufacture their own vaccines or lacked the resources for procurement.

Interpersonal Knowledge Gaps

Both Core and Multistakeholder GHD respondents confirmed gaps in GHD actors' lack of or insufficient knowledge around collaboration and teamwork. Global Health Diplomacy relies on bi-directional interpersonal interactions that may be internally facing (within one's immediate team or organization) or externally facing (between GHD actors and their counterparts). Thus, GHD actors need to know how to create or improve team coherence to improve efficiency and productivity. Core GHD actors emphasized GHD actors' knowledge gaps in bilateral and multilateral collaboration (Soherwordi, Qayyum, & Qayyum, 2022), especially in earlier stages of the pandemic, choosing to pursue individualistic interests instead. For Multistakeholder GHD actors, the lack of knowledge on team building prevented a more cohesive approach to GHD actors executing critical functions during the pandemic (Zapata, Buchnan & Azzopardi-Muscat, 2021).

Informal GHD actors did not mention interpersonal knowledge gaps regarding this theme. Considering interpersonal competencies were not mentioned by this group either, it can be inferred that respondents may have exhausted their recommendations while discussing interpersonal skills, for which they had earlier proposed a vast array of specific learned abilities. Alternatively, respondents may not have had any knowledge gaps in this area. They may also have perceived GHD actors' interpersonal abilities and their responses to each question as either mutually exclusive or as intersecting across the domains of knowledge, skills, or core competencies, thus excluding the need to reiterate their responses.

Technical Knowledge Gaps

Within this theme, Core, Multistakeholder, and Informal GHD actors underscored the need for training in specific technical or intricate areas, which, albeit diverse, reflected the diversity in GHD requirements. Core GHD actors mentioned the lack of knowledge of US foreign policy, global governance institutions, bilateral and multilateral negotiations, or how to navigate public health systems in host countries, amongst others. The role and responsibilities of a Core Global Health Diplomat are often underpinned by the knowledge of these specific domains, which may explain why these were flagged as important.

For Multistakeholder GHD actors, specific areas like how to conduct contact tracing or how to deal with passengers amid pandemic-imposed travel restrictions. Both of these examples were very specific to some of the functions the interviewees performed during the pandemic, for which they found themselves and their team members ill-equipped to handle.

For Informal GHD actors, intricate technical knowledge gap areas include leveraging the One Health approach (Mwatondo et al., 2023) in emergency responses, knowledge of risk management, public health policy and advocacy, and the Socioecological Model of Health, food production, climate change, and several more. These areas suggest a shift towards a systems-thinking approach to addressing global health challenges by considering the broader social and structural determinants of health that result in health disparities or inequitable access to healthcare.

Regarding more specific technical knowledge gaps, the Core and Informal GHD actor categories stated that GHD actors lacked knowledge of global health regulations, treaties, and instruments (Blinken & Becerra, 2021). Prior to the COVID-19 pandemic, there had been calls to ammend the International Health Regulations, which were last revised in 2005, in the wake of the SARS epidemic. The Core and Informal GHD actors also spotlighted a lack of understanding of performance frameworks or capacity assessments such as the Global Health Security Agenda's Joint External Evaluations (JEE). An understanding of these capacity assessments and Joint External Evaluations can help GHD actors assess the host country's preparedness and response capabilities to public health risks and identify gaps within the health system that need to be strengthened.

Among the Core GHD actors only, a strong emphasis was placed on GHD actors' lack of knowledge of supply chain management, which can shed light on the production, procurement, storage, delivery, and distribution of emergency supplies. This group also called out GHD actors' lack of clinical, global health, or public health expertise, which is vital for Global Health Diplomacy practice.

Both Multistakeholder and Informal GHD actors pointed out GHD actors' lack of familiarity with web communication technology such as Zoom and informatics in general (Gasparayan et al., 2021). This challenge could be explained by the fact that diplomatic interactions predominantly occur in person, and the relational aspects, nuances, and subtleties of these interactions cannot be replicated in a virtual space. Furthermore, these in-person engagements may have bypassed the need for GHD actors to use these communication applications prior to the pandemic, hence the lack of familiarity with this technology. Additionally, Multistakeholder GHD actors also mentioned GHD actors' lack of knowledge in several technical domains, including the understanding of the science underpinning the development of vaccines, diagnostics tests, and therapeutics, as well as epidemiology and statistics, which bore similarities to previous epidemic responses.

Critical and Analytical Thinking Knowledge Gaps

Core GHD respondents highlighted knowledge gaps in analytic and critical thinking expressed as GHD actors' inability to understand the limitations of scientific data in diagnostic, prevention, and therapeutic measures or how scientific inferences may evolve with new data. Furthermore, they noted a failure to understand and analyze emerging situations or priorities to know how and when to change course.

Informal GHD actors discussed GHD actors' lack of knowledge about public health ethics frameworks and how these can be applied to health interventions at the individual, community, and population levels (Hall-Clifford & Cook-Deegan, 2021). This understanding can provide guidance for GHD actors when implementing public health interventions or situations that pose moral or ethical dilemmas. For instance, how to make the determination for emergency use of the COVID-19 vaccine that had not undergone long-term clinical trials or deciding which priority population groups would receive the first doses of the vaccine whilst it was still unavailable to the wider public.

The Informal GHD actors also presented a lack of understanding of country governments' ability or commitment toward health interventions considering competing or 'more urgent' priorities. Additionally, the lack of a systems-based approach for assessing the implications of multisectoral global health issues may sometimes result in efforts to treat the symptoms of a health problem without fully understanding the root causes.

Multistakeholder GHD actors did not share any knowledge gaps related to the critical and analytical thinking theme. This theme also appeared to be missing from these participants' responses whilst discussing required core competencies for GHD practice. However, while discussing GHD actors' required skills, they mentioned the need for the ability to synthesize, analyze, and evaluate information objectively and logically to exercise sound judgment. This may mean that they either did not see any knowledge gaps pertaining to this theme or chose not to restate them, given their previous responses. It could also mean that this group of actors thought of knowledge, skills, and competencies as a continuum that aligns with the researcher's operating definition of core competencies as the proper application of knowledge, skills, and abilities at the right place and time.

Practical or Practice-Based Knowledge Gaps

While discussing gaps practice-based GHD knowledge gaps, Core GHD actors articulated the importance of having real-world experience from practicing Global Health Diplomacy and knowledge of donor requirements, including being results-driven and financially accountable for disbursed funding. Among the Multistakeholder GHD group, GHD actors need to understand that Global Health Diplomacy was not always fueled by altruism but could be employed for disruptive purposes (Fidler, 2021). For instance, the use of social media platforms to spread misinformation and disinformation or election interference, thereby undermining the public's trust in its elected officials or public health authority figures.

Informal GHD actors accentuated knowing how to engage and mobilize communities by identifying who the key GHD stakeholders are in specific contexts, as well as the knowledge of present and ongoing political and geopolitical shifts (Eurasia

Group, 2024) that would ultimately define GHD in a post-COVID era. For example, 2024 is a presidential election year in the United States. Whilst health has been recognized as a key foreign policy priority, at this time, it is unclear whether it will continue to garner bipartisan support or where it might fall on the incumbent president's foreign policy agenda. Conversely, there are other 'big issue' topics, such as the state of the economy and rising costs of living, immigration, or the uncontrolled use of artificial intelligence, that may take precedence over health.

For Core and Informal GHD actors, the knowledge of how to implement actual real-world pandemic responses, such as how to conduct lockdowns or social distancing measures, understanding the US emergency response system, and the responsibility of federal agencies in emergencies to mobilize, manage, and distribute finite resources was imperative (Moyazzem, Hossain, Abdulla, & Rahman, 2022). Multistakeholder and Informal GHD actors emphasized knowing how to lead during a crisis to mollify the polarization, chaos, and mistrust among populations witnessed during the COVID-19 pandemic (Abdi, Lega, & Ravagi, 2021).

Learning Knowledge Gaps

Core, Multistakeholder, and Informal GHD actors highlighted the inability to learn from the previous outbreaks or pandemics as a significant knowledge gap in all three groups of GHD actors (Talisuna et al., 2022; Juneau et al., 2022). The global challenges and inadequacies in the COVID-19 response reveal a lack of preparedness for global health emergencies. As a mitigation strategy, these GHD actors encouraged assessing countries' preparedness and response capacities and filling those gaps speedily and preemptively. One way to do this could be through training that utilizes simulation or tabletop exercises or using case studies where GHD actors could evaluate the strengths or weaknesses of a previous emergency response. Alternatively, the case studies may be used to elicit GHD actors' critical and analytical thinking by presenting them with emergency response scenarios and asking how they might respond under predefined circumstances.

Informal and Multistakeholder GHD actors also asserted the need for GHD actors to be willing and able to learn the technical requirements of their job, especially in emergencies, which require readiness, flexibility, and adaptability to the demands of the response (Taghizade, Chattu, Jaafaripooyan, & Kevany, 2021). Among the Core and Informal GHD actors, the lack of knowledge of how to deal with misinformation and disinformation and its impact on the credibility of public health practitioners, policymakers, and GHD actors themselves was also significant (Mutti, 2023). By and large, science and public health have been discredited and questioned in an unprecedented manner, which would require tremendous and consistent efforts to regain public trust. Concurrently, GHD actors, policymakers, and public health practitioners would also need to find new ways to rebuild the credibility of the global health and scientific community, and that of public health institutions like the World Health Organization.

Communication Knowledge Gaps

While discussing knowledge gaps related to communication, all actor categories emphasized GHD actors' lack of knowledge of how to communicate in emergencies. Emergency messaging, as seen in pandemic and outbreak responses, may contain information relevant to public health promotion, prevention, and protection to mitigate the loss of lives and property. Therefore, emergency communication should ideally be thoughtfully crafted and delivered in such a way that self-protective directives are clear, unambiguous, and easy to understand without undermining ongoing efforts toward the emergency response. Emergency communication should also be widely accessible and impress a sense of agency and trust in the target audience. It should also take into consideration potential barriers to adherence to recommendations based on individual or communal perceptions of susceptibility, severity, benefits, threats, and self-efficacy. Core and Informal GHD actors emphasized knowledge gaps in GHD actors' ability to access and share information promptly. They also questioned GHD actors' knowledge of how to properly frame public health messaging in an increasingly polarized society and mitigate the erosion of public trust. Core GHD actors furthermore discussed GHD actors' inadequacies around risk communication, which sometimes fails to identify and evaluate different levels of risk and develop measures to alleviate them. For Multistakeholder GHD respondents, the principal communication gaps were found in GHD actors' ability to communicate in emergencies and their lack of knowledge of foreign languages.

The table below presents an analysis of responses for required knowledge for GHD practice based on Core, Multistakeholder, and Informal GHD actors' responses to technical knowledge gaps. Areas, where a main theme was not mentioned in the GHD actors' responses, are left blank. The 'x' represents the GHD actors' responses corresponding to a specific sub-theme.

The technical knowledge requirements below reflect GHD actors' knowledge gaps in their roles and responsibilities during the COVID-19 pandemic and those recommended for GHD practice, now and in the future, depending on the functions they may be called to perform. For example, regarding similarities, all three GHD actor categories underscored the insufficiencies within the public health system expressed as a lack of public health resources and infrastructure, knowledge gaps in GHD actors' ability to learn from the past and communicate in emergency situations, and the need for GHD actors to be trained in diverse technical areas. Core and Multistakeholder GHD actors mentioned the need for GHD actors' knowledge of collaboration and teamwork, while Multistakeholder and Informal GHD actors emphasized the importance of GHD actors' knowledge of pandemic preparedness and response. Core and Informal stressed the need for GHD actors to know how to conduct lockdowns and social distancing measures.

On the other hand, some knowledge requirements are specifically featured within one GHD actor group and not in others. For example, the need for GHD actors to have clinical or public health experience for Core GHD actors, understanding how GHD can be used for disruptive or negative reasons for Multistakeholder GHD actors, or an understanding of politics and the geopolitical landscape for Informal GHD actors. However, this does not necessarily suggest that these knowledge requirements only pertain to the GHD actor group within which they were mentioned. The diversity in roles, functions, and responsibilities of GHD actors, as demonstrated by the recent pandemic, indicates the need for increased, broader, and targeted technical knowledge to ensure GHD actors are better equipped to practice GHD in a post-COVID era as their assignments continue to change and evolve.

Table 20

Data Analysis Table of Required Knowledge for Core, Multistakeholder, and Informal GHD Actors

RQ3 Knowledge				
Theme	Sub-theme	CORE	MSTK	INFML
Systemic	Public Health Resources and Infrastructure	x	x	x
	Human Resource or Staffing Gaps	x	x	

Category	Item			
	Limited Research and Publication in GHD Competencies	x		
	Pandemic Preparedness, Detection, and Response		x	x
	Data and Essential Resources Gaps			x
Interpersonal	Mix of interpersonal skills			None
	Collaboration and Teamwork	x	x	
Technical	Supply Chain Management	x		
	Clinical Global Health or Public Health Expertise	x		
	Understanding Global Health Instruments, Regulations & Treaties	x		x
	Performance Frameworks & Capacity Assessments	x		x
	Training in Intricate Technical Area	x	x	x
	Knowledge of Vaccines, Diagnostics & Therapeutics		x	
	Epidemiology and Statistics		x	
	Informatics/ Web Technology		x	x
Critical and Analytical Thinking			Lack of awareness of underlying principles: diagnostics, prevention measures, science behind vaccine development, limitations of scientific data. Being acquainted with ongoing and emerging issues	None	Public Health Ethics Frameworks, One Health, Lack of understanding of Gov's limitations on vaccine awareness, lack of understanding One Health and systems - thinking
Practical or Practice-Based	Practical or Real-World Global Health Diplomacy Experience	x		
	Understanding the US Emergency Response System	x		x
	Understanding Donor Requirements and Financial Accountability	x		
	Conducting Lockdowns and Social Distancing Measures	x		x
	Leadership		x	x
	Diplomacy for "wrong or unaltruistic" reasons		x	
	Community Engagement and Community Mobilization			x
	Understanding of Global Health Diplomacy stakeholders			x
	Understanding Politics and the Geopolitical Landscape			x
Learning	Ability to Learn from the Past	x	x	x
	On-the-job Learning		x	x
	Countering and Managing Misinformation and Disinformation	x		x
Communication	Access to Information and Knowledge Dissemination	x		x
	Communication in Emergencies	x	x	x
	Understanding Risk and Risk Communication	x		
	Erosion of Public Trust	x		x
	Foreign Language Gaps		x	

Aim 3: Define Global Health Diplomacy in a Post-COVID Era

Core GHD Actors' Definition of Global Health Diplomacy

The Core GHD actors' definition of Global Health Diplomacy recognizes the interconnectedness between population health and multiple sectors (Almeida, 2020), including economic development, education, national security, climate and the environment, and equity for marginalized groups (Gov.UK, 2021; Lee & Smith, 2011, p.1). Thus, it is incumbent on all policymakers in national and international forums to ensure health experts have a seat at the table when national security conversations are being had to ensure health is integrated into decision-making.

Global Health Diplomacy also provides a two-pronged approach to examining and addressing shared health challenges on a global scale (WHO.int, 2022) and finding solutions to complex health issues and trends that affect global institutions. The events of COVID-19 underscored the need for a more integrated and multisectoral approach to Global Health Diplomacy. This approach recognizes that health is always on the agenda. Health brings hope, and accessible, affordable, and equitable access to healthcare provides both a population safety net and greater economic output. However, it takes an amalgam of the right people or experts from various walks of life to ensure that health decisions are based on the best possible information and evidence. Ideally, this process should include people from the public and private sectors, from the grassroots or community level to the higher levels of policymaking (AlKhaldi et al., 2021).

Furthermore, the role of GHD actors for these respondents is also underpinned by cross-cultural collaborations, connections, and efforts amongst peer scientists and other stakeholders to foster programs, ideas, and objectives for a safer and healthier world

(OGA, 2023). Mirroring the requirements for specific expertise in politics, defense, culture, etc., for Foreign Service Officers assigned to American Embassies abroad, Core GHD actors should have health expertise, demonstrated by a health or clinical background, along with required technical skills to adequately represent the US' best global health interests.

Thus, the definition of Global Health Diplomacy by Core GHD actors also incorporates the diplomatic skills and competencies for advancing national interests and improving health outcomes (Fidler, 2013, p.693) through bilateral and multilateral communication, collaboration, and cooperation (Nkengasong, 2023). This process requires understanding foreign policy, global governance, scientific, technical, and development needs, assessing risk, and finding areas of agreement while mitigating conflict in diplomatic interactions amongst countries. For Global Health Diplomacy to be effective, GHD actors must appropriately apply the required knowledge, skills, and abilities for practice at the right place and time.

Multistakeholder Actors' Definition of Global Health Diplomacy

The definition of Global Health Diplomacy advanced by Multistakeholder GHD actors recognizes that current and future global health threats transcend international borders (Kickbusch et al., 2021). This state of flux of emerging disease outbreaks warrants a continuous state of preparedness and vigilance (Tahir et al., 2021), whether or not there's an active pandemic, and requires that GHD actors adopt a futuristic and proactive stance versus a reactive one toward addressing these threats (Baker et al., 2021).

These Multistakeholder GHD actors also recommended that health diplomacy engagements recognize the shift in bilateral and multilateral partnerships and interactions as the Global Health Diplomacy field evolves. Developing mutually beneficial partnerships (Bond, 2008, p.377) requires that actors genuinely inquire about the needs of their partners instead of assuming they have the answers or solutions. Global Health Diplomacy interactions are dependent on the level of engagement and the diversity of actors involved at the organizational, local, regional, national, and international levels. The level of interactions between these actors also calls for a deeper reflection on how the concept of GHD is being defined, calling for identifying areas of convergence of foreign policy and public health. Leveraging global health partnerships (Mahbubani, 2022) also facilitates a coordinated multistakeholder approach to improve domestic and multilateral communication and collaboration, strengthening global health security and safeguarding population health through global health investments (Gov.UK, 2021; Almeida, 2020).

Some of the GHD definitions provided by Multistakeholder GHD actors highlight the importance of community engagement and strengthening local capacity to support early detection and reporting of infectious disease outbreaks to contain their spread at the level at which they were identified (Bezbaruah et al., 2021). Essential to these efforts and aspirations is the importance of breaking down silos to build trusted relationships (Bond, 2008, p. 377) underpinned by technical collaborations and bi-directional learning (Weine et al., 2021), as well as the integration of scientific data to support evidence-based decision-making (Valz Gris et al., 2022).

Considering how the policies made within other sectors affect human health, the proposed definitions also highlight the need to move beyond human health towards a One Health approach to account for humanity's shared environment with plants and animals, environmental degradation, and climatic changes (Adisamito et al., 2022).

Informal Actors' Definition of Global Health Diplomacy

The Informal GHD actors' definition of Global Health Diplomacy also captures a diverse perspective that is both skills-based and dependent on the actors' engagements or interactions with other multilevel stakeholders (WHO.int, 2022). Some of these may involve discussions and dissemination of lessons learned or best practices in a post-COVID era. For these respondents, the definition of GHD was much more generalizable, where everyone who worked in global health or public health could potentially be a Global Health Diplomat.

For one Informal GHD actor the definition of GHD transcends the biomedical definition of health and incorporates multilevel, multistakeholder technical skills aimed at improving the well-being of humans on the planet, irrespective of where these actors were located. This definition highlighted the significant influence of political will, manifested through leaders' and policymakers' choices and decisions regarding individual and population health (PAHO, n.d.).

Other definitions embodied the understanding of the likelihood of imminent and future outbreaks, which required GHD actors to continuously acquire and develop skills and competencies to ensure they were prepared in the event of an epidemic (Kickbusch & Liu, 2022). These skills and competencies need not necessarily rest within government agencies like the CDC and USAID. Thus, Global Health Diplomacy skills can bridge the gap between medical and scientific innovation and implementation that leverage multistakeholder communication, cooperation, and collaboration to protect humanity's well-being during a future pandemic (Nkengasong, 2023).

However, one respondent felt defining GHD in a post-COVID era would be particularly challenging as any attempts to do so did not reflect the present-day reality of the geopolitical world in which we now live. Since foreign policy priorities and objectives define GHD efforts, GHD actors will be instructed on these foreign priorities and what resources are available for implementation. GHD definitions are often skewed towards Western democracies and hegemonic perceptions and fall short of considering the priorities or agendas of rising authoritarian regimes.

The Global Health Definitions advanced by Core, Multistakeholder, and Informal GHD actors appear to reflect their positionality, experience, roles and responsibilities, and their outlook of how they envision this field in a post-COVID era. While some of these definitions bear similarities to previous definitions presented in the literature review, there are some emerging concepts. For example, some definitions accentuated the integration of systems-thinking or leveraging the One Health approach, ensuring the GHD practice is science and evidence-based, as well as express consideration for population well-being instead of the biomedical definition of health. While these definitions are based on each actor's subjectivity, these actors all share one remarkable commonality: the COVID-19 pandemic was an unprecedented defining moment during which they practiced Global Health Diplomacy. As demonstrated by the literature, previous crucial moments in GHD history also called for the need to redefine this field that continues to evolve, perhaps accounting for why some definitions still refer to it as 'a nascent field.'

Considering the diversity in the roles of the GHD actors interviewed and the differences in how they defined GHD, it begs the question of whether each GHD actor category should have a separate definition of Global Health Diplomacy. If so, how might these new definitions account for the wide variety of actors in this field, taking into account the diversity of participants' responsibilities?

A synthesis of the proposed definitions showed similarities and differences across the Core, Multistakeholder, and Informal GHD actors. For example, the Core, Multistakeholder, and Informal GHD actors' definitions mentioned international collaboration with other GHD actors and the exchange of technical skills to solve health challenges. Multistakeholder and Informal GHD actors' definitions highlighted coordination for pandemic preparedness, the intersection of health and foreign policy, and its impact on population health outcomes. Informal and Multistakeholder GHD actors also noted the rapid spread of diseases and the need for proactive prevention efforts to strengthen health security. They also discussed leveraging One Health and recognizing and mitigating the effect of climate change on human health, food supply, and planetary sustainability. Core and Multistakeholder actors recognized the intricate link between health and other sectors, the need for a multisectoral approach to health decision-making, and the need to involve the community in identifying and reporting disease outbreaks.

Regarding differences, Informal GHD actors' definitions of GHD emphasized communication and negotiation with stakeholders, assessment of countries' health systems' capacity, collaborative approaches to identifying and addressing existing gaps, and understanding how foreign policy priorities and the changing geopolitical landscape will define the role of the GHD actors in a post-COVID era. Conversely, Core GHD actors recognized that health is always on the agenda and intersects with all other sectors, thus highlighting the need to build multilateral relationships and find areas of agreement while limiting areas of disagreement amongst countries. Multistakeholder GHD actors called for science and evidence-based GHD decisions and building partnerships to facilitate the exchange of ideas beyond the US to other countries.

A principal reason why GHD actors were asked to define GHD in a post-COVID era was to call for a reexamining of how previous definitions may have included or excluded the demands of a new era and how these definitions may inform current and future GHD practice. While the similarities and differences push past the boundaries of existing GHD definitions, the researcher recognizes that the post-COVID era is less than two years old. Therefore, it will require much more time for GHD actors to fully appraise all the requirements of a COVID-19 aftermath. The sample used for this study is also relatively small compared to the wider pool of GHD actors in each category. Thus, the proposed definitions cannot be generalized beyond this group as they may not accurately describe the sentiments of GHD actors who were not interviewed and whose perspectives are unaccounted for. Lastly, in view of the intersection between health and foreign policy and how foreign policy priorities often determine health priorities, many functions of GHD actors will be defined or influenced by policymakers' agenda-setting and decision-making. These aspects may potentially influence how these actors define Global Health Diplomacy.

Aim 4: Generate a summary of core competency requirements for GHD practice in a post-COVID era based on data from each GHD actor level.

This study provides new insights into the knowledge, skills, and core competencies of Core, Multistakeholder, and Informal Global Health Diplomacy actors. The similarities and differences within and between GHD actor groups for the themes earlier discussed are indicative of areas of convergence or divergence and not unanimity of GHD actors' responses.

The researcher set up the study aims and research questions to address specific study domains, knowledge (practical or theoretical understanding), skills (specific learned abilities), and core competencies (essential knowledge, skills, and abilities). This distinction was designed to facilitate an in-depth exploration of each domain to understand their requirements better and inform the development of GHD training.

A summary of specific Global Health Diplomacy core competencies was presented in Figure 5 in the previous chapter. An analysis of the core competencies from Core, Multistakeholder, and Informal GHD actors across the knowledge, skills, and competency domains revealed specific areas of convergence and divergence. For example, across the Core, Multistakeholder, and Informal GHD actors, GHD actors' ability to communicate knowledge and engagement of key stakeholders is deemed critical. Global Health Diplomacy is practiced by engaging with a diverse group of stakeholders across different settings and countries, which may explain why this core competency was proposed by all three actors.

Effective communication is also a key competency area for Core, Multistakeholder, and Informal GHD actors, who recommended that GHD actors be adequately trained in multiple communication formats, types, and mediums. Communication is the vehicle through which Global Health Diplomacy occurs. It underpins interactions between GHD actors, policymakers, and decision-makers, which may also explain why it is a core competency for each actor category. Core, Multistakeholder, and Informal GHD actors also underscored the need for training in specific technical or intricate areas, which varied significantly. Nevertheless, this divergence reflects the diversity in technical GHD requirements for each group of GHD actors and for each GHD actor interviewed. Similarly, the recommendations of the Global Health Diplomacy actors for practice-based competencies and their suggestions for training domains to enhance GHD practice were also remarkably diverse. This variance also reveals the multidisciplinary aspects of GHD demonstrated by the roles and responsibilities of GHD actors.

In general, the similarities and differences in core competencies within and between GHD actors indicate that the knowledge, skills, and core competencies requirements for GHD practice are not one-size-fits-all. Therefore, Global Health Diplomacy Training will need to be tailored to meet GHD actor's needs or the identified competency gaps. To effectively practice GHD or be considered competent, GHD actors must appropriately apply the required knowledge, skills, and abilities at the right place and time.

However, in practice, the findings suggest that GHD actors did not distinguish how and when they employed their knowledge, skills, and abilities. When discussing training, some GHD actors emphasized the need for clear professionalization pathways for public health and Global Health Diplomacy. At the end of 2022, there were calls for the creation of a US Foreign Health Service (Brown, 2022). While this advocacy was specific to Core GHD actors, the same argument can be made for the Multistakeholder and Informal GHD actors, using a tailored approach to build competency coupled with internships, externships, and mentorships for applied practice and real-world experience. Knowing and understanding the Essential Public Health functions was another strategic area highlighted in the training requirements of GHD actors, public health students, and health practitioners. However, only one respondent mentioned this. The World Health Organization defines Essential Public Health Functions as "the indispensable set of actions, under the primary responsibility of the state, that are fundamental for achieving the goal of public health, which is to improve, promote, protect, and restore the health of the population through collective action" (WHO.int, n.d.).

In real-world settings, global health diplomacy practice concurrently draws from an amalgam of knowledge, skills, and abilities at any given time. To practice GHD effectively or be considered competent, GHD actors will need to properly apply these knowledge, skills, and abilities at the right place and time. Respondents' awareness of the practical application of GHD may infer that their understanding of real-life practice requires that they employ their competencies (knowledge skills and abilities) in a non-distinct or overlapping manner. This explanation may account for why GHD actors may have mentioned specific learned abilities or traits when discussing required skills or why skills appear to have been 'omitted' when they spoke about competencies and vice versa. This explanation may also account for why the same specific learned abilities or traits may have been featured across two or all three study domains or why some study participants apologized 'for being repetitive' when responding to questions across domains and citing the same skill as a core competence or vice versa.

In the introductory chapter, the researcher highlighted two key studies that served as the foundation for her research, which are discussed below. The current study results build on existing evidence from the evaluation of US Health Attachés (Core GHD actors) profiles by Brown et al., 2018. Their study identified *"four main skills needed for successful GHD practice: diplomatic and negotiation skills, public health and scientific knowledge, an understanding of their Mission's overall priorities, and cross-cultural competency"* and other experiential skills from previous roles (Brown et al., 2018). Although the Health Attachés had mentioned learning on the job as the most efficient way to be trained for their roles, they also admitted not having received any training. Brown et al., 2018 also recommended standardized multidisciplinary training and mentorship opportunities for building skills in a practice-based setting, which aligns with this study's results. While the current study did not ask participants to distinguish between skills from previous roles, as some GHD actors reported their reliance on previous experience, just-in-time training, or team members' knowledge and expertise, this study has elicited a much more significant number of skills and competencies among the Core GHD or Health Attachés group. This could be explained by differences in the participants interviewed, which may also account for a difference in their roles, previous experience, or past and current responsibilities. Furthermore, the timing and timeline of the current study may also have drawn heavily from participants' recommendations of specific knowledge skills and competencies based on their lived experiences during the COVID-19 pandemic.

This study's results also built upon Katz et al., 2011 findings on defining Global Health Diplomacy in an era of globalization. Their study revealed that the *"expanding demands on global health diplomacy require a delicate combination of technical expertise, legal knowledge, and diplomatic skills that have not been systematically cultivated among either foreign service or global health professionals"* (Katz et al., 2011). The authors underlined the need to reassess the role of Global Health Diplomacy actors, as well as the skills, knowledge, and available resources for achieving health and foreign policy objectives. These recommendations are largely consistent with the responses and recommendations from the current study that call for required training to build and equip Global Health Diplomacy actors for a post-COVID era.

This research was meant to examine where Global Health Diplomacy Actors are and where they need to be in the post-COVID era. Throughout the pandemic and until now, public health has been politicized, polarized, and discredited, and science is being questioned in a way we have not seen before or were prepared for. While the Global Health Diplomacy taxonomy proposed by Katz et al., 2011 that classified GHD actors into Core, Multistakeholder, and Informal GHD actors is still relevant today, the current study results reveal several areas of overlap in the roles of all three GHD actor categories, as demonstrated by the summary of GHD core competencies. The findings revealed that during the COVID-19 pandemic, GHD actors were called upon to perform several new or different responsibilities, for which many were not equipped. These data also reflect the diverse responsibilities that GHD actors were called upon to execute in an emergency setting that fell outside the confines of their roles depicted by the GHD actor pyramid by Brown et al., 2014.

Considering the intersecting roles, priorities, goals, and responsibilities, the GHD taxonomy in a post-COVID era may be more appropriately represented by a three-circle Venn diagram depicting areas of convergence and divergence across all three GHD actor categories. Overall, these aspects reveal that Global Health Diplomacy has changed and will continue to evolve in this post-COVID era, given the changing foreign policy priorities and geopolitical landscape.

Figure 6
Global Health Diplomacy Actors in a Post-COVID Era

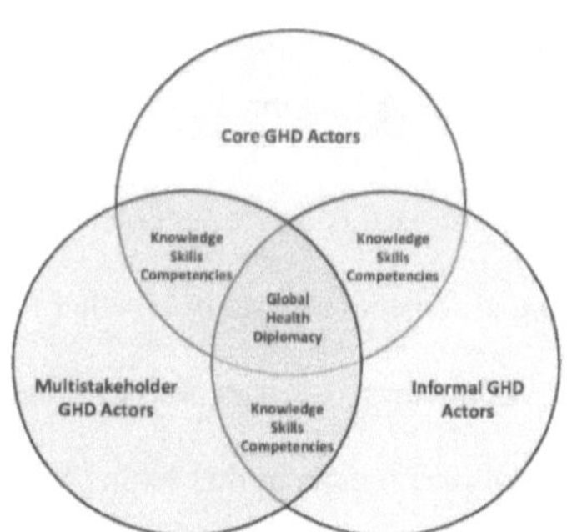

Implications for Policy and Recommendations

COVID-19 exposed significant gaps in Global Health Diplomacy actors' knowledge, skills, and competencies, which hindered their ability to respond effectively to a global pandemic. Significant diplomacy efforts occur through a whole-of-government and a whole-of-society approach and are imperative for strengthening early detection, global pandemic preparedness, and a coordinated response (State.gov., 2021). There is a compelling need to address these capacity gaps as other infectious diseases emerge while concurrently ensuring GHD actors are equipped to navigate and respond effectively to future health challenges (Van den Broucke, 2020).

On this premise, the Researcher proposes a novel conceptual framework, systematically developed by leveraging the literature review and integrating key informant interviews. This responsive conceptual framework reveals priority focus areas for Global Health Diplomacy in a post-COVID era. It proposes recommendations for strengthening the gaps and inadequacies of the pandemic response and challenges to practicing GHD during this period. It also represents a shift in how GHD actors' capacity and competency can be strengthened in a post-COVID world. This approach can concurrently strengthen global health security to ensure countries are better equipped to prevent, detect, and respond to global health threats speedily and comprehensively.

Conceptual frameworks are defined as "an interacting ecosystem that helps researchers intentionally bring all aspects of a study together through a process that explicates their connections, disjunctors, overlaps, tensions, and the context shaping a research setting and the study of phenomena in that setting" (Ravitch & Riggan, 2021, pg. 32). Conceptual frameworks can be used to underscore the relevance and significance of a research study (why the study matters), and how well the proposed design, data collection, and analysis are aligned to answer the research questions. They also help situate the research within theoretical and actual contexts and demonstrate how different framework components interact with each other (Ravitch & Riggan, 2016).

The proposed framework has seven main domains: health for diplomacy, bilateral and multilateral collaboration, surveillance and preparedness, strengthening systemic gaps, equitable access to healthcare, integrating health into all policies, and sustainable funding. Each domain is described in further detail below:

Health for Diplomacy: Strategically utilize health-related policies, initiatives, or interventions to advance diplomatic goals and achieve positive diplomatic outcomes through negotiations for conflict resolution, peace, sustainable development, economic stability, poverty reduction, social justice, and human rights.

Bilateral and Multilateral Collaboration: Leverage bilateral and multilateral diplomatic efforts and interactions to respond to global health threats, achieve global health objectives, and address health challenges for positive health outcomes, such as strengthening health systems and improving surveillance, data, and resource sharing.

Surveillance and Preparedness: Strengthen global health security through pandemic prevention, disease monitoring, data collection, analysis, interpretation, and sharing for evidence-based decision-making for early detection and rapid response.

Strengthening Systemic Gaps: Build and strengthen public health systems (workforce, infrastructure, financing, supply chains, diagnostics, and therapeutics) to respond to current and future health crises, including prevention and management of non-communicable diseases (NCDs), aging, and other emerging health needs.

Equitable Access to Healthcare: Address health inequities and structural and socioeconomic disparities to ensure accessible, affordable, and quality healthcare, as well as timely access to essential health services, vaccines, and treatment.

Integrating Health in all Policies: Advocate for One Health considerations at all levels of policy and decision-making by recognizing the influence of social, economic, climate, and environmental factors on health.

Sustainable Financing: Secure long-term funding for global health and global health security priorities, e.g., Health Systems Strengthening, research and development, and essential health service delivery.

Strengthening these priority domains is imperative in a post-COVID era, considering the high chances of another pandemic occurring and myriad threats to global health security. The diagram also represents the interconnectedness of each domain to the other six; for example, sustainable funding can ensure that health considerations are included in all policies. Negotiating global health policies and regulations requires bilateral and multilateral collaboration, which is essential to strengthening systemic gaps and preparing for, preventing, and responding to pandemics. International health negotiations and decision-making should be informed by evidence and anchored in principles of equity that eliminate disparities, making healthcare more accessible for marginalized populations. Global Health Diplomacy actors can also advocate for systematic health inequality monitoring, which requires countries to systematically collect and analyze qualitative and quantitative data (WHO.int, n.d.). Each of these domains is underpinned by GHD actors' proper application of their knowledge, skills, and abilities in interpersonal interactions, critical and analytical thinking, and communication.

Research has demonstrated significant benefits to population health outcomes when foreign policy goals and objectives align with those of health. Thus, health can be a soft power tool for proposing or developing an action plan and building consensus around a shared goal. This framework can also be applied to non-communicable diseases. Firstly, a root cause analysis should be performed to identify the causes of these health problems, followed by the collaborative development of contextualized solutions to address these diseases that significantly burden the health system and claim millions of lives yearly. Therefore, this novel conceptual framework proposes a holistic lens to enhance future Global Health Diplomacy policy, decision-making, and practice.

Figure 7
Global Health Diplomacy Priorities in a Post-COVID Era

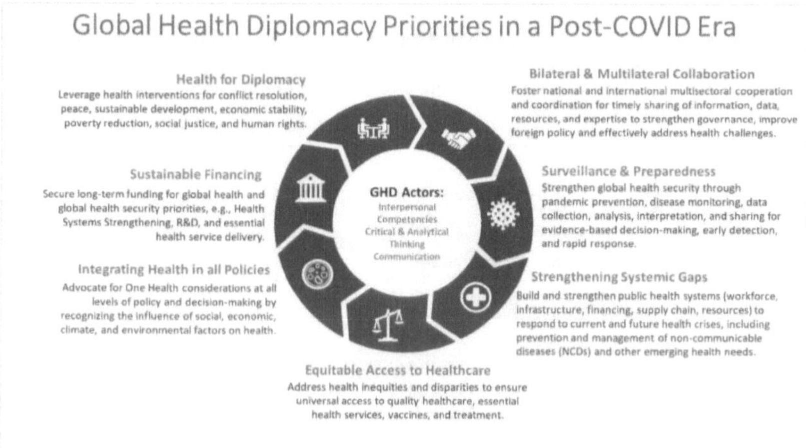

Implications for Practice and Recommendations

The study findings will inform the development of a training curriculum for current and future GHD actors or practitioners at Georgetown University's Health Diplomacy Training Institute. The GHD technical knowledge, skills, and core competencies proposed by study participants indicate potential training domains based on US GHD actors' perspectives and are in no way exhaustive. Considering the GHD

266

landscape in the post-COVID era is evolving, the Researcher anticipates that other training domains and priorities will continue to emerge, requiring tailoring the training curriculum accordingly (Yan & Saguine, 2021; UNESCO, 2020).

The Researcher also recognizes that current or prospective GHD actors may be at different proficiency levels and have different training requirements, which the Health Diplomacy Training Institute may want to explore further. For example, the NIH proficiency scale accounts for five levels of proficiency across each competency: "Fundamental Awareness (basic knowledge), Novice (limited experience), Intermediate (practical application), Advanced (applied theory), and Expert (recognized authority)" (NIH, 2017). Thus, the researcher recommends that the Health Diplomacy Training Institute conduct a needs assessment to ascertain the GHD actors' learning needs and objectives and to facilitate tailoring the training curriculum accordingly.

For training evaluation purposes, the Researcher recommends conducting pre-training and post-training assessments to infer the effect of the training on participants' knowledge. Depending on feasibility, the Researcher also suggests expansion of the training beyond the US either through a hybrid training model that allows for in-person and virtual participation or replication of the training in other regions to reach non-US-based GHD actors (Talisuna et al., 2022). The Researcher also acknowledges that specific simulation exercises may not mimic real-world GHD practice if training participants are not face-to-face.

Research Strengths and Limitations

This study contributes to understanding the knowledge, skills, and core competencies required by US Global Health Diplomacy actors in a post-pandemic era. The study also contributes to the research gap identified by the literature review: To the best of the Researcher's knowledge, no other study has explicitly focused on all three domains of required knowledge, skills, and core competencies for GHD practice across all three GHD actor categories. The study's exploratory, descriptive qualitative design and methodology, using semi-structured interviews, allowed for an in-depth exploration of each participant's perception of technical knowledge, skills, and core competencies for GHD practice.

The criterion sampling strategy may have potentially excluded pertinent key interested parties' viewpoints. For example, US GHD actors who may not be fluent in English or those who may not have access to the required technology or equipment for virtual interviews were not part of the study. Nevertheless, criterion sampling allowed this study to capture participants' rich perspectives that can still inform and improve current and future GHD practice. While study participants were grouped into three main categories, each participant's experience, perspective, and recommendation mirrored the uniqueness of their positionality within each actor category and the study. The study also revealed some similarities and differences in GHD actors' responses that may provide a better understanding of capacity strengthening or training initiatives.

The researcher also acknowledges the potential of researcher bias within the study, which can be manifested in her assumptions about the population being studied (Remler & Van Ryzin, 2015). To mitigate this issue, the Researcher strove to maintain reflexivity by reflecting on how her interaction with participants, personal beliefs, biases, and judgment may influence the interview process and/or the data being collected. While the Researcher is aware that qualitative data collection makes her an integral part of the research, she strove to pose interview questions to all participants in the same way. For investigator triangulation, the Researcher had an outside researcher and faculty member from the research committee review the initial interviews to provide feedback on the interviewing strategy, discuss challenges, and address potential biases.

Although the study population was confined to US GHD actors, many of these actors had international experience and cultural exposure from interacting with people from cultures within and outside of the US or from being stationed outside of the United States. These cross-cultural engagements may also have allowed them to draw from a broad range of experiences regarding required knowledge, skills, and core competencies (Biletska, Lastovskyi, & Semchynskyy, 2023). Therefore, although the research findings are informative, they are not meant to be generalizable to other GHD actors within and outside of the United States.

Lastly, the timing of the study also aligns with ongoing negotiations such as the Pandemic Agreement/Accord and amendment of International Health Regulations, which may impact the trajectory of future global health security and diplomacy priorities and the roles of GHD actors across all three groups. Also worthy of note is the Department of State's recent announcement establishing a Foreign Ministry Channel (FMC) on March 14, 2024 (State.gov, 2024). This initiative builds upon the 2022-2023 Global Action Plan for Enhanced Engagement (GAP) to elevate health as a national security priority. The FMC will have as primary objectives strengthening global health security by bolstering countries' pandemic prevention efforts and early-warning capacities; combatting

misinformation and disinformation in public health using technologies to strengthen

global health security, leveraging the One Health approach to mitigate the impact of

climate change on health, securing medical countermeasures for health emergencies, and

strengthening the capacity of diplomatic staff to respond to global health security threats

(State.gov., 2024).

Researcher Reflexivity

Throughout the research process, the researcher strove to reflect on how her lived

experiences, both personal and professional, and her 12-year career as a global health

practitioner could influence the research process. Practicing personal reflexivity required

that she assess how her values, beliefs, identity, and upbringing may affect data collection

and analysis decisions during the planning phase. The researcher used a journal to

document her feelings, thoughts, and reactions to help her identify her biases or

assumptions coming into the study and how they might have changed over time. These

memos also included her recall of the events surrounding the COVID-19 pandemic and

her assessment of the US pandemic response.

During the interview process, the researcher consciously reminded herself that her

role as the interviewer was that of a doctoral candidate conducting research, not a global

health diplomacy actor or global health professional. This stance allowed her to ask

questions and listen without influencing participants' responses. While her professional

background may have allowed for more comfortable interactions with interview

participants, she refrained from inadvertently being pulled into the discussion. The

researcher also took notes during the interview and wrote down her initial thoughts immediately after each interview to document things participants shared that surprised her, including thematic outliers. She also kept memos of emerging salient themes during the transcript-cleaning process. Memoing helped document her interactions with participants and the data, supported the generation of themes and ideas, and guided data interpretation, thus improving research credibility.

Implications for Future Research

The scope of this research study principally focused on US Global Health Diplomacy actors. While the 21 study participants offered rich, insightful, and informative perspectives into their lived experiences and practice of GHD, the Researcher acknowledges they are a subset of the broader pool of GHD actors in different parts of the world. Thus, further research may explore knowledge, skills, and competencies for GHD practice on other continents, juxtaposed against this study's findings, to inform GHD policy and practice in the country or context in which the research is conducted. Furthermore, this study did not include participants from authoritarian states or non-democracies, whose perspectives are integral in understanding GHD democracy in a post-COVID era rife with geopolitical tensions, or their impression of GHD practice by countries considered democracies.

Conclusion

Humanity constantly faces global health challenges of varying proportions, many of which require international coordination and collaboration. Even as countries struggle to recover from the far-reaching consequences of the COVID-19 pandemic, the question of where the next global health threat emerges looms large. The impacts of climate change, infectious disease outbreaks, reemerging diseases, and antimicrobial resistance are some of the main priorities.

There is growing recognition of the importance of effective preparedness and prevention and the ability to rapidly detect and respond to global health threats. Global Health Diplomacy is central to facilitating and assuring global prevention, preparedness, and response efforts to imminent health threats with immediacy and intentionality. Therefore, strengthening Global Health Diplomacy requires GHD actors to have the proper knowledge, skills, and core competencies to navigate the intersection of public health and foreign policy priorities to build partnerships that foster a collective approach to addressing health threats with immediacy and intentionality.

References

Abdi, Z., Lega, F., Ebeid, N., & Ravaghi, H. (2021). Role of hospital leadership in combating the COVID-19 pandemic. *Health Services Management Research, 35*(1), 2–6.

Africa CDC. (2019). Our History. Retrieved from https://africacdc.org/about-us/our-history/

Alilio, M., Hariharan, N., Lugten, E., Garrison, K., Bright, R., Owembabazi, W., … Saldana, K. (2022). Strategies to Promote Health System Strengthening and Global Health Security at the Subnational Level in a World Changed by COVID-19. *Global Health: Science and Practice, 10*(2), e2100478.

AlKhaldi, M., James, N., Chattu, V. K., Ahmed, S., Meghari, H., Kaiser, K., … Tanner, M. (2021). Rethinking and strengthening the Global Health Diplomacy through triangulated nexus between policy makers, scientists and the community in light of COVID-19 global crisis. *Global Health Research and Policy, 6*(1).

Adams, V., Novotny, T. E., & Leslie, H. (2008). Global Health Diplomacy. *Medical Anthropology, 27*(4), 315–323.

Adisasmito, W. B., Almuhairi, S., Behravesh, C. B., Bilivogui, P., Bukachi, S. A., Casas, N., … Zhou, L. (2022). One health: A new definition for a sustainable and Healthy Future. *PLOS Pathogens, 18*(6). doi:10.1371/journal.ppat.1010537

Alegbeleye, B. J., & Mohammed, R. K. (2020). Challenges of healthcare delivery in the context of COVID-19 pandemic in Sub-Saharan Africa. *Iberoamerican Journal of Medicine, 2*(2), 100–109.

Alhojailan, M. I. (2012). Thematic Analysis: A Critical Review of its Process and Evaluation. Retrieved from https://www.westeastinstitute.com/wp-content/uploads/2012/10/ZG12-191-Mohammed-Ibrahim-Alhojailan-Full-Paper.pdf

Almeida, C. (2020, February 28). Global Health Diplomacy: A Theoretical and Analytical Review.

Ariansen, A. M., Gloppen, S., Rakner, L., Johansson, K. A., & Haaland, Ø. A. (2020). Time for Global Health Diplomacy. *The Lancet, 395*(10238), 1691–1692. doi:10.1016/s0140-6736(20)30490-6

Asadi-Lari, M., Ahmadi Teymourlouy, A., Maleki, M., & Afshari, M. (2021). Opportunities and challenges of global health diplomacy for prevention and control of noncommunicable diseases: a systematic review. *BMC Health Services Research, 21*(1).

AU.int. (n.d.). AU in a Nutshell. Retrieved from https://au.int/en/au-nutshell

Baker, R. E., Mahmud, A. S., Miller, I. F., Rajeev, M., Rasambainarivo, F., Rice, B. L., … Metcalf, C. J. (2021). Infectious disease in an ERA of global change. *Nature Reviews Microbiology, 20*(4), 193–205. doi:10.1038/s41579-021-00639-z

Barber, C. (2023). COVID-19 v. Flu: A "much more serious threat," new study into long-term risks concludes. Retrieved from https://fortune.com/2023/12/14/COVID-19-v-flu-more-serious-threat-new-study-health-carolyn-barber/

Bauer, M. S., Damschroder, L., Hagedorn, H., Smith, J., & Kilbourne, A. M. (2015). An introduction to implementation science for the non-specialist. *BMC Psychology, 3*(1). doi:10.1186/s40359-015-0089-9

Bayati, M., Noroozi, R., Ghanbari-Jahromi, M., & Jalali, F. S. (2022). Inequality in the distribution of COVID-19 vaccine: A systematic review. *International Journal for Equity in Health, 21*(1). doi:10.1186/s12939-022-01729-x

Berlinguer G. (1999). Globalization and global health. *International journal of health services : planning, administration, evaluation, 29*(3), 579–595. https://doi.org/10.2190/1P5R-QV3M-2YHH-JN3F

Bernard, H. R., Wutich, A., & Ryan, G. W. (2017). *Analyzing qualitative data: Systematic approaches* (2nd ed.). Thousand Oaks etc.: SAGE.

Bezbaruah, S., Wallace, P., Zakoji, M., Padmini Perera, W. S., & Kato, M. (2021). Roles of community health workers in advancing health security and resilient health systems: emerging lessons from the COVID-19 response in the South-East Asia Region. *WHO South-East Asia Journal of Public Health, 10*(3), 41.

Biddle, L., Wahedi, K., & Bozorgmehr, K. (2020). Health system resilience: a literature review of empirical research. *Health policy and planning, 35*(8), 1084–1109. https://doi.org/10.1093/heapol/czaa032

Biletska, O., Lastovskyi, V., & Semchynskyy, K. (2023). Intercultural Economic and Communication Competence: International Relations and Diplomacy Area. *Economic Affairs, 68*(1s). doi:10.46852/0424-2513.1s.2023.20

Bishop F. L. (2015). Using mixed methods research designs in health psychology: an illustrated discussion from a pragmatist perspective. *British journal of health psychology*, *20*(1), 5–20. https://doi.org/10.1111/bjhp.12122

Blau, F., Koebe, J., & Meyerhofer, P. (2020). Who are the essential and frontline workers? *National Bureau of Economics Research*. doi:10.3386/w27791

Blinken, A. (2023). Press Statement: Launch of the Bureau of Global Health Security and Diplomacy. Retrieved from https://www.state.gov/launch-of-the-bureau-of-global-health-security-and-diplomacy/

Blinken, A., & Becerra, X. (2021). Strengthening Global Health Security and reforming the International Health Regulations. *JAMA*, *326*(13), 1255. doi:10.1001/jama.2021.15611

Bollyky, T. J., & Patrick, S. M. (2020). The U.S. must learn from COVID-19 to prevent the next disaster. Retrieved from https://www.cfr.org/report/pandemic-preparedness-lessons-COVID-19

Boro, E., & Stoll, B. (2022). Barriers to COVID-19 health products in low-and middle-income countries during the COVID-19 pandemic: A rapid systematic review and evidence synthesis. *Frontiers in Public Health*, *10*. doi:10.3389/fpubh.2022.928065

Boujnah, H. (2022). Health diplomacy in Africa-opportunities post-COVID-19. *Pan African Medical Journal, 43*.

Bourgeault, I. L., Maier, C. B., Dieleman, M., Ball, J., MacKenzie, A., Nancarrow, S., … Sidat, M. (2020). The COVID-19 pandemic presents an opportunity to develop more sustainable health workforces. *Human Resources for Health, 18*(1).

Bradshaw, C., Atkinson, S., & Doody, O. (2017). Employing a Qualitative Description Approach in Health Care Research. *Global qualitative nursing research*, *4*, 2333393617742282. https://doi.org/10.1177/2333393617742282

Brown, M. (2022). The United States Needs a Foreign Health Service. Retrieved from https://www.thinkglobalhealth.org/article/united-states-needs-foreign-health-service

Brown, M. D., Bergmann, J. N., Novotny, T. E., & Mackey, T. K. (2018). Applied global health diplomacy: profile of health diplomats accredited to the UNITED STATES and foreign governments. *Globalization and health, 14*(1), 2. https://doi.org/10.1186/s12992-017-0316-7

Brown, M., Mackey, T., Shapiro, C., Kolker, J., & Novotny, T. (2014). Bridging Public Health and Foreign Affairs: The Tradecraft of Global Health Diplomacy and the Role of Health Attachés. Retrieved from https://www.sciencediplomacy.org/sites/default/files/bridging_public_health_and_f oreign_affairs_science__diplomacy.pdf

Burau, V., Falkenbach, M., Neri, S., Peckham, S., Wallenburg, I., & Kuhlmann, E. (2022). Health system resilience and health workforce capacities: Comparing health system responses during the COVID19 pandemic in six European countries. *The International Journal of Health Planning and Management, 37*(4), 2032–2048.

Busetto, L., Wick, W., & Gumbinger, C. (2020). How to use and assess qualitative research methods. Retrieved from https://neurolrespract.biomedcentral.com/articles/10.1186/s42466-020-00059-z

CARPHA. (2022). Who we are. Retrieved from https://carpha.org/Who-We-Are/About

Carter, H. H., & Bollyky, T. J. (2024). Global Health Security and Diplomacy in 2024: Lead, leverage, and elevate: Think global health. Retrieved from https://www.thinkglobalhealth.org/article/global-health-security-and-diplomacy-2024-lead-leverage-and-elevate

CDC Office of Policy, Performance, and Evaluation. (2022). Retrieved from https://www.cdc.gov/policy/polaris/policyprocess/policyanalysis/index.html#:~:text =Policy%20Analysis%20is%20the%20process,%2C%20efficient%2C%20and%20 feasible%20one.

CDC.gov. (2022-a). Timeline of CDC's Global Health Milestones from 1942-2021. Retrieved from https://www.cdc.gov/globalhealth/resources/reports/annual/2022/timeline.html

CDC.gov. (2022-b). What is the Global Health Security Agenda? Retrieved from https://www.cdc.gov/globalhealth/security/what-is-ghsa.htm

CDC.gov. (2022-c). CDC - about CDC's public health ethics activities - OSI - OS. Retrieved from https://www.cdc.gov/os/integrity/phethics/index.htm

CDC.gov. (2023-a). COVID Data Tracker. Retrieved from https://COVID.cdc.gov/COVID-data-tracker/#trends_weeklydeaths_select_00

CDC.gov. (2023-b). One health basics. Retrieved from
    https://www.cdc.gov/onehealth/basics/index.html#:~:text=What%20is%20One%20
    Health%3F,more%20important%20in%20recent%20years.

CDC.gov. (2024). CDC COVID Data tracker. Retrieved from
    https://covid.cdc.gov/covid-data-
    tracker/#trends_weeklyhospitaladmissions_select_00

Center for Global Health Science and Security. (2023). Health Diplomacy Training
    Institute. Retrieved from https://ghss.georgetown.edu/health-diplomacy-training-
    institute/

CFR. (2017). Tools of foreign policy: What is Diplomacy? Retrieved from
    https://world101.cfr.org/foreign-policy/tools-foreign-policy/what-diplomacy

CFR. (2023). A brief history of U.S. foreign aid. Retrieved from
    https://world101.cfr.org/global-era-issues/development/brief-history-us-foreign-aid

CGD. (2021). What's Next? Predicting The Frequency and Scale of Future Pandemics.
    Retrieved from https://www.cgdev.org/event/whats-next-predicting-frequency-and-
    scale-future-pandemics

Chafe R. (2017). The Value of Qualitative Description in Health Services and Policy
    Research. Valeur de la description qualitative dans la recherche sur les politiques et
    services de santé. *Healthcare policy = Politiques de sante*, *12*(3), 12–18.

Chattu, V. (2017). The rise of Global Health Diplomacy: An interdisciplinary concept
    linking health and international relations. *Indian Journal of Public Health*, *61*(2),
    134. doi:10.4103/ijph.ijph_67_16

Chen, Q., Rodewald, L., Lai, S., & Gao, G. F. (2021). Rapid and sustained containment
    of COVID-19 is achievable and worthwhile: Implications for pandemic response.
    BMJ. doi:10.1136/bmj-2021-066169

Clingendael. (2021). Global Health Training For Diplomats: A Tailor Made Toolkit.
    Retrieved from https://www.clingendael.org/news/global-health-training-
    diplomats-tailor-made-toolkit

Council of American Ambassadors. (n.d.). American Diplomacy and the Foreign
    Language Challenge. Retrieved from
    https://www.americanambassadors.org/publications/ambassadors-review/fall-
    2008/american-diplomacy-and-the-foreign-language-challenge

Cullinan, K. (2023). IHR negotiations to continue until May 2024. Retrieved from
     https://healthpolicy-watch.news/ihr-negotiations-to-continue-until-may-
     2024/#:~:text=Negotiations%20at%20the%20World%20Health,as%20far%20as%2
     0May%202024.

Czabanowska, K., & Kuhlmann, E. (2021). Building back better after COVID-19: public
     health competencies for health workforce preparedness. *European Journal of
     Public Health, 31*(Supplement_3).

Czyzewski, K. (2011). Colonialism as a broader social determinant of health.
     International Indigenous Policy Journal, 2(1). doi:10.18584/iipj.2011.2.1.5

Dalla Lana School of Public Health. (2023). Executive Course in Global Health
     Diplomacy. Retrieved from https://www.dlsph.utoronto.ca/institutes/centre-for-
     global-health/global-health-diplomacy-course/

Danaa, S. (2023). Introduction to the whole-of-government approach. Retrieved from
     https://unosd.un.org/sites/unosd.un.org/files/session_10-2_mr._samuel_danaa.pdf

Daniel, A. (2023). The world hopes to enact a pandemic treaty by May 2024. will it
     succeed or flail? Retrieved from
     https://www.npr.org/sections/goatsandsoda/2023/09/21/1200816304/the-world-
     hopes-to-enact-a-pandemic-treaty-by-may-2024-will-it-succeed-or-flail

Davison, C. M., Bartels, S. A., Purkey, E., Neely, A. H., Bisung, E., Collier, A., …
     Adams, L. V. (2021). Last mile research: A conceptual map. *Global Health Action,
     14*(1). doi:10.1080/16549716.2021.1893026

de Quadros, C. A., & Epstein, D. (2002). Health as a bridge for peace: PAHO's
     experience. *The Lancet, 360.* doi:10.1016/s0140-6736(02)11808-3

Dedoose. (n.d.). Home: Great Research Made Easy. Retrieved from
     https://www.dedoose.com/

DeVine, M. E. (2020). Intelligence Community Support to pandemic preparedness …
     Retrieved from https://crsreports.congress.gov/product/pdf/IF/IF11537

Dhami, S., Thompson, D., El Akoum, M., Bates, D. W., Bertollini, R., & Sheikh, A.
     (2022). Data-enabled responses to pandemics: Policy lessons from COVID-19.
     Nature Medicine, 28(11), 2243–2246. doi:10.1038/s41591-022-02054-0

Ding, D., & Zhang, R. (2022). China's COVID-19 control strategy and its impact on the global pandemic. *Frontiers in Public Health, 10*. doi:10.3389/fpubh.2022.857003

Diplo. (2023). Health Diplomacy. Retrieved from https://www.diplomacy.edu/topics/health-diplomacy/#:~:text=International%20Organizations%3A%20Operating%20in%20the,crucial%20role%20in%20health%20diplomacy.

DOD. (2020). Operation warp speed official: First COVID-19 vaccines to arrive Monday. Retrieved from https://www.defense.gov/News/News-Stories/Article/Article/2445137/operation-warp-speed-official-first-COVID-19-vaccines-to-arrive-monday/

DOD. (2023). Memorandum for Senior Pentagon Leadership Commanders of the Combatant Commands Defense Agency and DOD Field Activity Directors. Retrieved from https://media.defense.gov/2023/Jan/31/2003153299/-1/-1/1/MEMORANDUM-CONSOLIDATED-DEPARTMENT-OF-DEFENSE-CORONAVIRUS-DISEASE-2019-FORCE-HEALTH-PROTECTION-GUIDANCE-REVISION-4.PDF

Dubb, S. S. (2020). Coronavirus pandemic: Applying a whole-of-society model for the whole-of-the world. *British Journal of Oral and Maxillofacial Surgery, 58*(7), 838–842. doi:10.1016/j.bjoms.2020.05.009

ECDC. (2017). About ECDC. Retrieved from https://www.ecdc.europa.eu/en/about-ecdc

Elm Learning. (2023). Microlearning. Retrieved from https://elmlearning.com/hub/elearning/microlearning/

Elman, C., Gerring, J., Mahoney, J., & Swedberg, R. (2020). Chapter 2: Exploratory Research. In *The production of knowledge: Enhancing progress in social science* (pp. 17–41). Cambridge, United Kingdom: Cambridge University Press.

ElSayed, D. O. (2020). Health Diplomacy As A Soft Power: What COVID-19 Has Taught Us. 6(6), 11–20.

EPA. (2021). Understanding the Connections Between Climate Change and Human Health. Retrieved from https://www.epa.gov/climate-indicators/understanding-connections-between-climate-change-and-human-health

Eurasia Group. (2024). Eurasia group: The top risks of 2024. Retrieved from https://www.eurasiagroup.net/issues/top-risks-2024

European Commission. (2022). International Organisations and Multilateral fora. Retrieved from https://digital-strategy.ec.europa.eu/en/policies/international-organisations

FA.gov. (n.d.). ForeignAssistance.gov Dashboard 2022. Retrieved from https://www.foreignassistance.gov/

Faizullaev, A. (2014). Diplomatic interactions and negotiations. *Negotiation Journal, 30*(3), 275–299. doi:10.1111/nejo.12061

Fauci, A. S. (2022). It ain't over till it's over…but it's never over — emerging and reemerging infectious diseases. *New England Journal of Medicine, 387*(22), 2009–2011. doi:10.1056/nejmp2213814

Faustino, R., Faria, M., Teixeira, M., Palavra, F., Sargento, P., & do Céu Costa, M. (2022). Systematic Review and meta-analysis of the prevalence of coronavirus: One health approach for a global strategy. *One Health, 14*, 100383. doi:10.1016/j.onehlt.2022.100383

Feldbaum, H., Lee, K., & Michaud, J. (2010). Global health and foreign policy. Epidemiologic reviews, 32(1), 82–92. https://doi.org/10.1093/epirev/mxq006

FEMA. (2020). Coronavirus (COVID-19) pandemic: National Resource Prioritization Cell. Retrieved from https://www.fema.gov/fact-sheet/coronavirus-COVID-19-pandemic-national-resource-prioritization-cell

Fidler, D. (2001). The globalization of public health: the first 100 years of international health diplomacy. *Bulletin of the World Health Organization.*

Fidler, D. (2010). The Challenges of Global Health Governance. Retrieved from https://www.sadil.ws/bitstream/handle/123456789/160/Challenges-of-Global-Health-Governance.pdf?sequence=1&isAllowed=y

Fidler, D. (2011). Rise and Fall of Global Health as a Foreign Policy Issue1. Retrieved from https://www.ghgj.org/DavidFidler.pdf

Fidler, D. P. (2020). The COVID-19 pandemic, geopolitics, and international law. *Journal of International Humanitarian Legal Studies, 11*(2), 237–248. doi:10.1163/18781527-bja10010

Fidler, D. P. (2021). Global Health's reckoning with realpolitik: Think global health. Retrieved from https://www.thinkglobalhealth.org/article/global-healths-reckoning-realpolitik

Frenk, J., Gómez-Dantés, O., & Moon, S. (2014). From sovereignty to Solidarity: A renewed concept of global health for an ERA of complex interdependence. *The Lancet, 383*(9911), 94–97. doi:10.1016/s0140-6736(13)62561-1

Frutos, R., Gavotte, L., Serra-Cobo, J., Chen, T., & Devaux, C. (2021). COVID-19 and emerging infectious diseases: The Society is still unprepared for the next pandemic. *Environmental Research, 202*, 111676. doi:10.1016/j.envres.2021.111676

Galvão, J. (2023). COVID-19: Forgetting a pandemic that is not over. *The Lancet, 401*(10386), 1422–1423. doi:10.1016/s0140-6736(23)00637-2

Gasparyan, A. Y., Kumar, A. B., Yessirkepov, M., Zimba, O., Nurmashev, B., & Kitas, G. D. (2022). Global Health Strategies in the Face of the COVID-19 Pandemic and Other Unprecedented Threats. *Journal of Korean Medical Science, 37*(22).

Gauttam, P., Singh, B., & Kaur, J. (2020). COVID-19 and Chinese Global Health Diplomacy: Geopolitical Opportunity for China\textquoterights Hegemony? *Millennial Asia, 11*(3), 318–340.

Geneva Graduate Institute. (2024). Training. Retrieved from https://www.graduateinstitute.ch/research-centres/global-health-centre/training

GHSA. (2023). A partnership against global health threats. Retrieved from https://globalhealthsecurityagenda.org/

Ginsbach, K., Monahan, J., & Gottschalk, K. (2021). Beyond COVID-19: Reimagining the role of International Health Regulations in the Global Health Law Landscape. Retrieved from https://www.healthaffairs.org/content/forefront/beyond-COVID-19-reimagining-role-international-health-regulations-global-health-law

Glaser, B. G. (1965). The constant comparative method of qualitative analysis. *Social Problems, 12*(4), 436–445. doi:10.1525/sp.1965.12.4.03a00070

Glaser, B. G., & Strauss, A. L. (2017). The discovery of Grounded Theory: Strategies for qualitative research (Version PDF). *George Mason Library Catalog* (First). Londres: Routledge. Retrieved from https://wrlc-gm.primo.exlibrisgroup.com/discovery/fulldisplay?docid=alma9947481480704105&context=L&vid=01WRLC_GML:01WRLC_GML&lang=en&search_scope=MyInst_and_CI&adaptor=Local%20Search%20Engine&isFrbr=true&tab=Everything&query=any,contains,253912&sortby=date_d&facet=frbrgroupid,include,26559772750717368&offset=0

Gostin, L. O., & Katz, R. (2016). The International Health Regulations: The governing framework for global health security. Retrieved from https://www.ncbi.nlm.nih.gov/pmc/articles/PMC4911720/

GOV.UK. (2021). Characteristics of global health diplomacy. Retrieved from https://www.gov.uk/research-for-development-outputs/characteristics-of-global-health-diplomacy

Green, J., Thorogood, N., Green, J., & Thorogood, N. (2018). Chapter 10: Beginning Data Analysis. In *Qualitative Methods for Health Research* (4th ed., pp. 258–262). London, UK: SAGE PUBLICATIONS.

Green, L., Ashton, K., Bellis, M. A., Clemens, T., & Douglas, M. (2021). 'health in all policies'—a key driver for health and well-being in a post-COVID-19 Pandemic World. *International Journal of Environmental Research and Public Health*, *18*(18), 9468. doi:10.3390/ijerph18189468

Guterres, A. (2021). Press Release: Vaccine nationalism, hoarding putting us all at risk, secretary-general tells World Health Summit, warning COVID-19 will not be last global pandemic | UN press. Retrieved from https://press.un.org/en/2021/sgsm20986.doc.htm

GWU Office of Human Research. (n.d.). Retrieved from https://humanresearch.gwu.edu/reviewtypes

Haines, J. (2024). Countries that receive the most foreign aid from the U.S. | best ... Retrieved from https://www.usnews.com/news/best-countries/articles/countries-that-receive-the-most-foreign-aid-from-the-u-s

Hajira Arif. (2021). UN Peacekeeping during Health Crises: COVID-19 and Expansion of Mission Mandates. *NUST Journal of International Peace & Stability*, 113–118.

Haldane, V., De Foo, C., Abdalla, S. M., Jung, A.-S., Tan, M., Wu, S., … Legido-Quigley, H. (2021). Health Systems Resilience in managing the COVID-19 pandemic: Lessons from 28 countries. *Nature Medicine*, *27*(6), 964–980. doi:10.1038/s41591-021-01381-y

Hall-Clifford, R., & Cook-Deegan, R. (2021). Ethically managing risks in global health fieldwork: Human rights ideals confront real world challenges. Retrieved from https://www.hhrjournal.org/2019/06/ethically-managing-risks-in-global-health-fieldwork-human-rights-ideals-confront-real-world-challenges/

Hall-Clifford, R., & Cook-Deegan, R. (2021). Ethically managing risks in global health fieldwork: Human rights ideals confront real world challenges. Retrieved from https://www.hhrjournal.org/2019/06/ethically-managing-risks-in-global-health-fieldwork-human-rights-ideals-confront-real-world-challenges/

Health.gov. (n.d.). Poverty. Retrieved from https://health.gov/healthypeople/priority-areas/social-determinants-health/literature-summaries/poverty

Healthy People 2030. (n.d.). Social Determinants of Health. Retrieved from https://health.gov/healthypeople/priority-areas/social-determinants-health

HHS.gov. (2023). Fact Sheet: End of the COVID-19 Public Health Emergency. Retrieved from https://www.hhs.gov/about/news/2023/05/09/fact-sheet-end-of-the-COVID-19-public-health-emergency.html

HHS.gov. (n.d.). From the Factory to the Frontlines The Operation Warp Speed Strategy for Distributing a COVID-19 Vaccine. Retrieved from https://www.hhs.gov/sites/default/files/strategy-for-distributing-COVID-19-vaccine.pdf

History.State.gov. (n.d.). MILESTONES: 1914–1920 The League of Nations, 1920. Retrieved from https://history.state.gov/milestones/1914-1920/league

Hoffman, S. J. (10 2010). Strengthening global health diplomacy in Canada's foreign policy architecture: Literature review and key informant interviews. *Canadian Foreign Policy Journal, 16*(3), 17–41.

Hotez, P. J. (2014). ``Vaccine Diplomacy'': Historical Perspectives and Future Directions. *PLoS Neglected Tropical Diseases, 8*(6), e2808.

IOM. (2009). A prominent role for health in U.S. foreign policy - the US ... Retrieved from https://www.ncbi.nlm.nih.gov/books/NBK32621/

ITC. (2023). The role of diplomacy in facilitating International Trade. Retrieved from https://thetradecouncil.com/the-role-of-diplomacy-in-facilitating-international-trade/

Jahn, B., Friedrich, S., Behnke, J., Engel, J., Garczarek, U., Münnich, R., ... Friede, T. (2022). On the role of data, statistics and decisions in a pandemic. *AStA Advances in Statistical Analysis, 106*(3), 349–382. doi:10.1007/s10182-022-00439-7

Javed, S., & Chattu, V. K. (2020). Strengthening the COVID-19 pandemic response, global leadership, and international cooperation through global health diplomacy. *Health Promotion Perspectives, 10*(4), 300–305.

Jeggo, M., Arabena, K., & Mackenzie, J. S. (2019). One health and global security into the future. *One Planet, One Health*, 21–52. doi:10.2307/j.ctvggx2kn.7

Jenkins, B. M. (2023). Pandemics don't really end-they echo. Retrieved from https://time.com/6307629/COVID-19-pandemic-over-essay/

Jones, L., & Hameiri, S. (2022). Explaining the failure of global health governance during COVID-19. *International Affairs*, 98(6), 2057–2076. doi:10.1093/ia/iiac231

Jørgensen, F., Bor, A., Rasmussen, M. S., Lindholt, M. F., & Petersen, M. B. (2022). Pandemic fatigue fueled political discontent during the COVID-19 pandemic. *Proceedings of the National Academy of Sciences, 119*(48). doi:10.1073/pnas.2201266119

Juneau, C.-E., Pueyo, T., Bell, M., Gee, G., Collazzo, P., & Potvin, L. (2022). Lessons from past pandemics: A systematic review of evidence-based, cost-effective interventions to suppress COVID-19. *Systematic Reviews, 11*(1). doi:10.1186/s13643-022-01958-9

Katz, R., Kornblet, S., Arnold, G., Lief, E., & Fischer, J. E. (2011). Defining health diplomacy: changing demands in the era of globalization. *The Milbank quarterly, 89*(3), 503–523. https://doi.org/10.1111/j.1468-0009.2011.00637.x

Kaye, A. D., Okeagu, C. N., Pham, A. D., Silva, R. A., Hurley, J. J., Arron, B. L., … Cornett, E. M. (2021). Economic impact of COVID-19 pandemic on healthcare facilities and systems: International Perspectives. *Best Practice & Research Clinical Anaesthesiology, 35*(3), 293–306. doi:10.1016/j.bpa.2020.11.009

Kevany, S. (2016). Global health engagement in diplomacy, intelligence and counterterrorism: a system of standards. *Journal of Policing, Intelligence and Counter Terrorism, 11*(1), 84–92.

KFF. (2022). Retrieved from https://www.kff.org/global-health-policy/fact-sheet/the-u-s-government-and-global-health/

KFF. (2023). Breaking down the U.S. Global Health Budget by program area. Retrieved from https://www.kff.org/global-health-policy/fact-sheet/breaking-down-the-u-s-global-health-budget-by-program-

area/#:~:text=In%20FY%202023%2C%20funding%20for%20global%20health%2
0totaled%20%2412.9%20billion.

Khullar, D., & Chokshi, D. (2018). Health, Income, & Poverty: Where We Are & What Could Help. Retrieved from https://www.healthaffairs.org/do/10.1377/hpb20180817.901935/

Kickbusch, I. (2007). Global health diplomacy: the need for new perspectives, strategic approaches and skills in global health. *Bulletin of the World Health Organization, 85*(3), 230–232.

Kickbusch, I., & Buss, P. (9 2011). Global Health Diplomacy and Peace. *Infectious Disease Clinics of North America, 25*(3), 601–610.

Kickbusch, I., & Liu, A. (2022). Global health diplomacy—reconstructing power and governance. *The Lancet, 399*(10341), 2156–2166. doi:10.1016/s0140-6736(22)00583-9

Kickbusch, I., & Liu, A. (2022). Global health diplomacy—reconstructing power and governance. *The Lancet, 399*(10341), 2156–2166. doi:10.1016/s0140-6736(22)00583-9

Kickbusch, I., Behrendt, T., Di Ruggiero, E., Gong, J., Karaman, E., Michaelides, O., & Watulo, F. (2021). Global health diplomacy. Retrieved from https://www.oxfordbibliographies.com/display/document/obo-9780199756797/obo-9780199756797-0101.xml

Kickbusch, I., Ivanova, M. (2013). The History and Evolution of Global Health Diplomacy. In: Kickbusch, I., Lister, G., Told, M., Drager, N. (eds) Global Health Diplomacy. *Springer, New York, NY.* https://doi.org/10.1007/978-1-4614-5401-4_2

Kickbusch, I., Nikogosian, H., Kazatchkine, M., & Kokeny, M. (2021). Retrieved from https://www.graduateinstitute.ch/sites/internet/files/2021-02/GHC-Guide.pdf

Kickbusch, I., Silberschmidt, G., & Buss, P. (2007). Retrieved from https://www.ncbi.nlm.nih.gov/pmc/articles/PMC2636243/

Kim, D. J., & Kim, A. I. (5 2022). Global health diplomacy and North Korea in the COVID-19 era. *International Affairs, 98*(3), 915–932.

Kim, H., Sefcik, J. S., & Bradway, C. (2017). Characteristics of Qualitative Descriptive Studies: A Systematic Review. *Research in nursing & health, 40*(1), 23–42. https://doi.org/10.1002/nur.21768

Kingdon, J. W. (1995). The Policy Primevial Soup/Criteria for survival. In *Agendas, alternatives, and public policies* (2nd ed., pp. 131–143). essay, New York, NY: HarperCollins College Publishers.

Koplan, J. P., Bond, T. C., Merson, M. H., Reddy, K. S., Rodriguez, M. H., Sewankambo, N. K., & Wasserheit, J. N. (2009). Towards a common definition of global health. *The Lancet, 373*(9679), 1993–1995. doi:10.1016/s0140-6736(09)60332-9

Kristen Jogerst, Brian Callender, Virginia Adams, Jessica Evert, Elise Fields, Thomas Hall, … Lynda L Wilson. (2015). Identifying interprofessional global health competencies for 21st-century health professionals. *Annals of Global Health.*

Kuhlmann, E., Dussault, G., & Correia, T. (5 2021). Global health and health workforce development: what to learn from COVID19 on health workforce preparedness and resilience. *The International Journal of Health Planning and Management, 36*(S1), 5–8.

Lazzarini, I. (2015). The forms of diplomatic communication. *Communication and Conflict*, 188–212. doi:10.1093/acprof:oso/9780198727415.003.0011

Ledford, H. (2022). COVID vaccine hoarding might have cost more than a million lives. *Nature*. doi:10.1038/d41586-022-03529-3

Lefrançois, T., Malvy, D., Atlani-Duault, L., Benamouzig, D., Druais, P.-L., Yazdanpanah, Y., … Lina, B. (2023). After 2 years of the COVID-19 pandemic, translating one health into action is urgent. *The Lancet, 401*(10378), 789–794. doi:10.1016/s0140-6736(22)01840-2

Leite, D. F. B., Padilha, M. A. S., & Cecatti, J. G. (2019). Approaching literature review for academic purposes: The Literature Review Checklist. Retrieved from https://www.ncbi.nlm.nih.gov/pmc/articles/PMC6862708/

Levin-Zamir, D., Sorensen, K., Su, T. T., Sentell, T., Rowlands, G., Messer, M., … Okan, O. (2021). Health promotion preparedness for health crises -- a \textquoteleftmust\textquoteright or \textquoteleftnice to have\textquoteright? Case studies and global lessons learned from the COVID-19 pandemic. *Global Health Promotion, 28*(2), 27–37.

Levy, B. (2002). Health and peace. Retrieved from
    https://pubmed.ncbi.nlm.nih.gov/11885034/

Lewandowsky, S., Linden, S. van der, & Norman, A. (2024). Disinformation is the real
    threat to democracy and public health. Retrieved from
    https://www.scientificamerican.com/article/disinformation-is-the-real-threat-to-
    democracy-and-public-health/

Lister, G., & Lee, K. (2012). The Process and Practice of Negotiation. Global Health
    Diplomacy: Concepts, Issues, Actors, Instruments, Fora and Cases, 73–87.
    https://doi.org/10.1007/978-1-4614-5401-4_6

Lister, G., & Told, M. (2012). Current and Future Issues in Global Health Diplomacy. In
    Global Health Diplomacy (pp. 27–36). *Springer New York.*

Luh, S., & Baltag, D. (2021). The role of EU health attachés for global health diplomacy
    in times of COVID-19. *Global Affairs, 7*(6), 903–920.

Maani, N., Abdalla, S. M., Ettman, C. K., Parsey, L., Rhule, E., Allotey, P., & Galea, S.
    (2023). Global Health Equity requires global equity. *Health Equity, 7*(1), 192–196.
    doi:10.1089/heq.2022.0169

Mackenzie, J. S. (n.d). The WHO response to SARS and preparations for the future.
    Retrieved from https://www.ncbi.nlm.nih.gov/books/NBK92476/

Mac-Seing, M., Gidey, M., & Ruggiero, E. D. (2023). COVID-19-related global health
    governance and Population Health Priorities for health equity in G20 countries: A
    scoping review. *International Journal for Equity in Health, 22*(1).
    doi:10.1186/s12939-023-02045-8

Mahbubani, K. (2022). Multilateral Diplomacy. In: The Asian 21st Century. China and
    Globalization. *Springer, Singapore.* https://doi.org/10.1007/978-981-16-6811-1_43

Marani, M., Katul, G. G., Pan, W. K., & Parolari, A. J. (2021). Intensity and frequency of
    extreme novel epidemics. *Proceedings of the National Academy of Sciences,
    118*(35). doi:10.1073/pnas.2105482118

Martin, E., Nolte, I., & Vitolo, E. (2016). The four Cs of Disaster Partnering:
    Communication, Cooperation, coordination and collaboration. *Disasters, 40*(4),
    621–643. doi:10.1111/disa.12173

Meerts, P. W. (2015). Chapter 10. In *Diplomatic negotiation: Essence and evolution* (pp. 243–268). The Hague: Clingendael Institute.

Michaud, J., & Kates, J. (2013). Global health diplomacy: Advancing foreign policy and global health interests. *Global Health: Science and Practice, 1*(1), 24–28. doi:10.9745/ghsp-d-12-00048

Milani, F. (2020). COVID-19 outbreak, social response, and early economic effects: A global VAR analysis of cross-country interdependencies. *Journal of Population Economics, 34*(1), 223–252. doi:10.1007/s00148-020-00792-4

Moore, C. (2023). BRICS and global health diplomacy in the COVID-19 pandemic: Situating Brics' diplomacy within the prevailing global health governance context. Retrieved from https://www.redalyc.org/journal/358/35872854011/html/

Moyazzem, H. M., Abdulla, F., & Rahman, A. (2022). Challenges and difficulties faced in low- and middle-income countries during COVID-19. *Health Policy OPEN, 3*, 100082. doi:10.1016/j.hpopen.2022.100082

Moyer, J. D., Verhagen, W., Mapes, B., Bohl, D. K., Xiong, Y., Yang, V., … Hughes, B. B. (2022). How many people is the COVID-19 pandemic pushing into poverty? A long-term forecast to 2050 with alternative scenarios. *PLOS ONE, 17*(7). doi:10.1371/journal.pone.0270846

Mutti A. (2023). From Pandemic to World Instability and War Crimes: Lessons Learned in a Turbulent Socio-Political Landscape. *La Medicina del lavoro, 114*(6), e2023052. https://doi.org/10.23749/mdl.v114i6.15436

Mwatondo, A., Rahman-Shepherd, A., Hollmann, L., Chiossi, S., Maina, J., Kurup, K. K., … Dar, O. (2023). A global analysis of one health networks and the proliferation of one health collaborations. *The Lancet, 401*(10376), 605–616. doi:10.1016/s0140-6736(22)01596-3

Naderifar, M., Goli, H., & Ghaljaie, F. (2017). Snowball sampling: A purposeful method of sampling in qualitative research. *Strides in Development of Medical Education, 14*(3). doi:10.5812/sdme.67670

NARA. (2020). Coronavirus Response. Retrieved from https://trumpwhitehouse.archives.gov/issues/coronavirus/

NCCC. (n.d.). Curricula enhancement module series. Retrieved from https://nccc.georgetown.edu/curricula/culturalcompetence.html#:~:text=Cultural%2

0competence%20is%20a%20set,effectively%20in%20cross%2Dcultural%20situati
ons.

Neergaard, M. A., Olesen, F., Andersen, R. S., & Sondergaard, J. (2009). Qualitative
description - the poor cousin of health research?. *BMC medical research
methodology, 9*, 52. https://doi.org/10.1186/1471-2288-9-52

NIH. (2017). What is the NIH proficiency scale? Retrieved from
https://hr.nih.gov/about/faq/working-nih/competencies/what-nih-proficiency-scale

Nkengasong, J. (2023). Retrieved from https://oversight.house.gov/wp-
content/uploads/2023/12/20231206-AMB-Nkengasong-Select-COVID-
Subcommittee-1213-Hearing-Testimony-vOMB_Cleared.pdf

Novotny, T. E., Kickbusch, I., & Told, M. (2013). 21st Century Global Health
Diplomacy. WORLD SCIENTIFIC.

Nye, J. (2017). Soft power: The origins and political progress of a concept. *Palgrave
Communications, 3*(1). doi:10.1057/palcomms.2017.8

Odell, J., & Tingley, D. (n.d.). Negotiating Agreements in International Relations.
Retrieved from
https://www.apsanet.org/portals/54/Files/Task%20Force%20Reports/Chapter7Man
sbridge.pdf

ODNI. (2021). Global Trends 2040. Retrieved from
https://www.dni.gov/index.php/gt2040-home/keythemes

OECD. (2023). The United States' whole-of-government approach to global health ...
Retrieved from https://www.oecd.org/development-cooperation-
learning/practices/the-united-states-whole-of-government-approach-to-global-
health-challenges-ed48d383/

Office of Foreign Assistance. (2021). About US – office of foreign assistance - united
states department of state. Retrieved from https://www.state.gov/about-us-office-of-
foreign-assistance/

OGA. (2021). Why HHS Works Globally. Retrieved from
https://www.hhs.gov/about/agencies/oga/about-oga/why-hhs-works-
globally/index.html

OGA. (2022). Health Attachés. Retrieved from
https://www.hhs.gov/about/agencies/oga/global-health-diplomacy/health-attaches/index.html

OGA. (2023-a). Global health diplomacy. Retrieved from
https://www.hhs.gov/about/agencies/oga/global-health-diplomacy/index.html

OGA. (2023-b). Office of Global Affairs: Multilateral Relations Office. Retrieved from
https://www.hhs.gov/about/agencies/oga/about-oga/what-we-do/international-relations-division/multilateral-relations.html

One Health Commission. (2022). What is One Health? Retrieved from
https://www.onehealthcommission.org/en/why_one_health/what_is_one_health/

PAHO. (n.d.). History of PAHO. Retrieved from https://www.paho.org/en/who-we-are/history-paho

PAHO. (n.d.). What is Health Diplomacy and why important & relevant.pdf. Retrieved
from https://www.paho.org/spc-crb/dmdocuments/What is Health Diplomacy and
Why Important & Relevant.pdf

Pancheshnikov, A., Cuneo, C. N., Matias, W. R., Cázares-Adame, R., Santos López, A.
G., Paxton, R. M., & Chen, C. C. G. (4 2023). Case studies in adaptation: centring
equity in global health education during the COVID-19 pandemic and beyond. *BMJ
Global Health, 8*(4), e011682.

Patton, M. Q. (2015). Purposeful sampling. In *Qualitative Evaluation and research
methods. Second edition* (pp. 169–186). Newbury Park Calif: Sage.

Payne, C. B. (2021). Global Health Engagement: Leveraging New Technology and
Multilateral Partnerships During the COVID-19 Pandemic. *Military Medicine,
187*(1–2), 4–6.

Ramanadhan, S., Revette, A. C., Lee, R. M., & Aveling, E. L. (2021). Pragmatic
approaches to analyzing qualitative data for implementation science: An
introduction. *Implementation Science Communications, 2*(1). doi:10.1186/s43058-021-00174-1

Ramirez-Rubio, O., Daher, C., Fanjul, G., Gascon, M., Mueller, N., Pajín, L., …
Nieuwenhuijsen, M. J. (2019). Urban health: An example of a "health in all
policies" approach in the context of sdgs implementation - *Globalization and
Health*. Retrieved from

https://globalizationandhealth.biomedcentral.com/articles/10.1186/s12992-019-0529-z

Ravitch, S., & Riggan, M. (2021). Conceptual Frameworks in Research. Retrieved from https://us.sagepub.com/sites/default/files/upm-assets/110533_book_item_110533.pdf

Reina Ortiz, M., Sharma, V., Casanova, J., Corvin, J., & Hoare, I. (2021). Developing global health diplomacy-related skills using a COVID-19-like epidemic simulation as a learning strategy. *The American Journal of Tropical Medicine and Hygiene*, *105*(1), 59–65. doi:10.4269/ajtmh.21-0155

Remler, D. K., & Van Ryzin, G. G. (2015). Research Methods in Practice: Strategies for Description and Causation. Retrieved from https://edge.sagepub.com/remler3e

Rhee, K., Crabtree, C., & Horiuchi, Y. (2023). Perceived motives of public diplomacy influence foreign public opinion. *Perceived Motives of Public Diplomacy Influence Foreign Public Opinion*. doi:10.1007/s11109-022-09849-4

Rodriguez-Garcia, R., Macinko, J., Solorzano, F. X., & Schlesser, M. (2001). How can health serve as a bridge for peace? Certi crisis ... Retrieved from https://hsrc.himmelfarb.gwu.edu/cgi/viewcontent.cgi?article=1227&context=sphhs_global_facpubs

Roser, M., Ritchie, H., & Spooner, F. (2021). Burden of disease. Retrieved from https://ourworldindata.org/burden-of-disease#:~:text=We%20see%20strong%20differentiation%2C%20with,in%20the%20Central%20African%20Republic.

Ruckert, A., Labonté, R., Lencucha, R., Runnels, V., & Gagnon, M. (2016). Global health diplomacy: A critical review of the literature. *Social Science & Medicine*, *155*, 61–72. doi:10.1016/j.socscimed.2016.03.004

Rudolph, L., Caplan, J., Ben-Moshe, K., & Dillon, L. (2013). Health in All Policies: A Guide for State and Local Governments. Washington, DC and Oakland, CA: American Public Health Association and Public Health Institute.

Rungius, C., & Flink, T. (2020). Romancing science for global solutions: On narratives and interpretative schemas of science diplomacy. *Humanities and Social Sciences Communications*, *7*(1). doi:10.1057/s41599-020-00585-w

Sandelowski M. (2010). What's in a name? Qualitative description revisited. *Research in nursing & health*, *33*(1), 77–84. https://doi.org/10.1002/nur.20362

Schmidt, A. (2023). Health and peace: The future of international emergency health responses during violent conflict. Retrieved from https://www.ipinst.org/2023/10/health-and-peace-the-future-of-international-emergency-health-responses-during-violent-conflict

Sending, O. J., Pouliot, V., & Neumann, I. B. (2011). The future of diplomacy: Changing practices, evolving relationships. *International Journal, 66*(3), 527–542. http://www.jstor.org/stable/23104366

Shrestha, N., Shad, M. Y., Ulvi, O., Khan, M. H., Karamehic-Muratovic, A., Nguyen, U.-S. D. T., … Haque, U. (2020). The impact of COVID-19 on globalization. Retrieved from https://www.ncbi.nlm.nih.gov/pmc/articles/PMC7553059/

Sirleaf, E. J., & Clark, H. (2021). Report of the Independent Panel for Pandemic Preparedness and response: Making COVID-19 the last pandemic. *The Lancet, 398*(10295), 101–103. doi:10.1016/s0140-6736(21)01095-3

Skidmore, S. (2022). Exploratory Research | Definition, Purpose & Examples. Retrieved from https://study.com/learn/lesson/research-types-examples-exploratory-descriptive-explanatory.html

Smith, R., & Hanson, K. (2011). Global health diplomacy: the 'missing pillar' of health system strengthening. In *Oxford Academic* (Online). essay, Oxford.

Soherwordi, S. H., Qayyum, S., & Qayyum, F. (2022). Multilateralism and human security: Situating the nature and scope of "global health diplomacy" (GHD) in the context of covid19. *NUST Journal of International Peace & Stability.* doi:10.37540/njips.v5i2.134

State.gov. (2021). Retrieved from https://www.state.gov/key-topics-office-of-international-health-and-biodefense/using-a-whole-of-government-approach-to-advance-health-objectives/

State.gov. (2022). Plans for a Bureau of Global Health Security and Diplomacy. Retrieved from https://www.state.gov/plans-for-a-bureau-of-global-health-security-and-diplomacy/

State.gov. (2023-a). About Us – PEPFAR - United States Department of State. Retrieved from https://www.state.gov/about-us-pepfar/

State.gov. (2023-b). Bureau of Global Health Security and diplomacy - united states department of state. Retrieved from https://www.state.gov/bureaus-offices/secretary-of-state/bureau-of-global-health-security-and-diplomacy/

State.gov. (2023-c). Launch of the Bureau of Global Health Security and diplomacy - united states department of state. Retrieved from https://www.state.gov/launch-of-the-bureau-of-global-health-security-and-diplomacy/

State.gov. (2023-d). John N. Nkengasong - United States Department of State. Retrieved from https://www.state.gov/biographies/john-n-nkengasong/

State.gov. (2023-e). COVID-19 response and Recovery - United States Department of State. Retrieved from https://www.state.gov/COVID-19-recovery/

State.gov. (2024). State Department announces New Lateral Entry Pilot Program - United States Department of State. Retrieved from https://www.state.gov/state-department-announces-new-lateral-entry-pilot-program/

State.gov. (2024). United States hosts launch of Foreign Ministry Channel for Global ... Retrieved from https://www.state.gov/united-states-hosts-launch-of-foreign-ministry-channel-for-global-health-security/

Stoto, M. A., Schlageter, S., & Kraemer, J. D. (2022). COVID-19 mortality in the United States: It's been two Americas from the start. *PLOS ONE, 17*(4). doi:10.1371/journal.pone.0265053

Taghizade, S., Chattu, V. K., Jaafaripooyan, E., & Kevany, S. (2021). Covid-19 pandemic as an excellent opportunity for Global Health Diplomacy. *Frontiers in Public Health, 9.* doi:10.3389/fpubh.2021.655021

Tagliabue, F., Galassi, L., & Mariani, P. (2020). The "Pandemic" of Disinformation in COVID-19. *SN comprehensive clinical medicine, 2*(9), 1287–1289. https://doi.org/10.1007/s42399-020-00439-1

Tago, A. (2017). Multilateralism, bilateralism, and unilateralism in foreign policy. *Oxford Research Encyclopedia of Politics.* doi:10.1093/acrefore/9780190228637.013.449

Tahir, M. J., Sawal, I., Essar, M. Y., Jabbar, A., Ullah, I., & Ahmed, A. (2021). Disease X: A hidden but inevitable creeping danger. *Infection Control & Hospital Epidemiology, 43*(11), 1758–1759. doi:10.1017/ice.2021.342

Talisuna, A. O., Bonkoungou, B., Mosha, F. S., Struminger, B. B., Lehmer, J., Arora, S., ... Moeti, M. R. (2020). The COVID-19 pandemic: Broad Partnerships for the rapid scale up of innovative virtual approaches for capacity building and credible information dissemination in Africa. *Pan African Medical Journal, 37.* doi:10.11604/pamj.2020.37.255.23787

Taylor, L. (2024). Who pandemic treaty: "Torrent of fake news" has put negotiations at risk, says who chief. Retrieved from https://www.bmj.com/content/384/bmj.q243

The World Bank. (2023). The pandemic fund. Retrieved from https://fiftrustee.worldbank.org/en/about/unit/dfi/fiftrustee/fund-detail/pppr

Thomas, M. D. (n.d.). ODNI releases declassified assessment on COVID-19 origins. Retrieved from https://www.intelligence.gov/publics-daily-brief/public-s-daily-brief-articles/1089-odni-releases-declassified-assessment-on-COVID-19-origins

Torner, N. (2023). The end of COVID-19 public health emergency of international concern (PHEIC): And now what? *Vacunas (English Edition)*, *24*(3), 164–165. doi:10.1016/j.vacune.2023.05.001

Tulchinsky, T. H., & Varavikova, E. A. (2014). A History of Public Health. *The New Public Health*, 1–42. https://doi.org/10.1016/B978-0-12-415766-8.00001-X

UN.org. (2012). Taking a whole- of-government approach - public institutions. Retrieved from https://publicadministration.un.org/egovkb/Portals/egovkb/Documents/un/2012-Survey/Chapter-3-Taking-a-whole-of-government-approach.pdf

UN.org. (2015). Universal Declaration of Human Rights. Retrieved from https://www.un.org/en/udhrbook/pdf/udhr_booklet_en_web.pdf

UN.org. (2020). COVID-19 Impacting Global Security with Heightened Volatility, Increased Threats to United Nations Personnel, Secretary-General Says in New Report. Retrieved from https://press.un.org/en/2020/org1711.doc.htm

UN.org. (2023-a). WHO chief declares end to COVID-19 as a global health emergency. Retrieved from https://news.un.org/en/story/2023/05/1136367

UN.org. (2023-b). Zero-draft-PPPR-political-declaration-5-june.PDF. Retrieved from https://www.un.org/pga/77/wp-content/uploads/sites/105/2023/06/Zero-draft-PPPR-Political-Declaration-5-June.pdf

UN.org. (n.d.). The 17 Goals. Retrieved from https://sdgs.un.org/goals

UNESCO. (2020). Education in a post-COVID world: Nine ideas for public action. Retrieved from https://en.unesco.org/sites/default/files/education_in_a_post-COVID_world-nine_ideas_for_public_action.pdf

UNGeneva.org. (n.d.). The League of Nations. Retrieved from
https://www.ungeneva.org/en/about/league-of-nations/overview

USAID.gov. (2022-a). Joint Strategic Plan FY 2022 – 2026. Retrieved from
https://www.usaid.gov/sites/default/files/2022-05/Final_State-USAID_FY_2022-
2026_Joint_Strategic_Plan_29MAR2022.pdf

USAID.gov. (2022-b). Where we work. Retrieved from https://www.usaid.gov/where-
we-work

USAID.gov. (2023-a). Global Health Security: Protecting the World from Health
Emergencies. Retrieved from https://www.usaid.gov/global-health/health-
areas/global-health-security

USAID.gov. (2023-b). Mission, Vision, and Values. Retrieved from
https://www.usaid.gov/about-us/mission-vision-values

USAID.gov. (2023-c). United States announces $250 million planned contribution to the
Pandemic Fund to support pandemic prevention, preparedness, and Response: Press
Release. Retrieved from https://www.usaid.gov/news-information/press-
releases/may-19-2023-united-states-announces-250-million-planned-contribution-
pandemic-fund-support-pandemic-prevention-preparedness-and-response

USDA.gov. (n.d.). Coronavirus disease (COVID-19). Retrieved from
https://www.usda.gov/coronavirus

Valz Gris, A., Gualano, M. R., Osti, T., Villani, L., Corona, V. F., D'ambrosio, F., …
Ricciardi, W. (2022). Leadership in public health crisis: a review to summarize
lessons learned from COVID-19 pandemic. *European Journal of Public Health,
32*(Supplement_3).

Van den Broucke, S. (2020). Why health promotion matters to the COVID-19 pandemic,
and vice versa. *Health Promotion International, 35*(2), 181–186.

Vériter, S. L., Bjola, C., & Koops, J. A. (2020). Tackling covid-19 disinformation:
Internal and external challenges for the European Union. *The Hague Journal of
Diplomacy, 15*(4), 569–582. doi:10.1163/1871191x-bja10046

VoA. (2024). Building Stronger Health Security in 2024. Retrieved from
https://editorials.voa.gov/a/building-stronger-health-security-in-2024/7437413.html

Volle, A. (2023, November 29). *Globalization. Encyclopedia Britannica.*
https://www.britannica.com/money/topic/globalization

Voss, J., Yasobant, S., Akridge, A., Tarimo, E., Seloilwe, E., Hausner, D., & Mashalla,
Y. (2021). Gaps, Challenges, and Opportunities for Global Health Leadership
Training. *Annals of Global Health, 87*(1), 62. https://doi.org/10.5334/aogh.3219

Vuković, S. (2020). The many faces of power in diplomatic negotiations. *SAIS Review of
International Affairs, 40*(1), 45–57. doi:10.1353/sais.2020.0004

WEF. (2023). Climate change is adding to a growing infectious disease burden – we need
coordinated action now. Retrieved from
https://www.weforum.org/agenda/2023/01/climate-change-is-adding-to-a-growing-
infectious-disease-burden-our-healthcare-systems-need-coordinated-action-now/

Weine, S., Bosland, M., Rao, C., Edison, M., Ansong, D., Chamberlain, S., &
Binagwaho, A. (2021). Global Health Education Amidst COVID-19: Disruptions
and Opportunities. *Annals of Global Health, 87*(1), 12.

Weiner, S. (2020). The new coronavirus affects us all. But some groups may suffer more.
Retrieved from https://www.aamc.org/news/new-coronavirus-affects-us-all-some-
groups-may-suffer-more

White House.gov. (2023). Fact sheet: Biden-Harris Administration Releases Global
Health Security Partnerships Annual Progress Report demonstrating results from
United States Investments. Retrieved from https://www.whitehouse.gov/briefing-
room/statements-releases/2023/12/30/fact-sheet-biden-%E2%81%A0harris-
administration-releases-global-health-security-partnerships-annual-progress-report-
demonstrating-results-from-united-states-investments/

Whiteside, R. (2008). American diplomacy and the Foreign Language Challenge.
Retrieved from https://www.americanambassadors.org/publications/ambassadors-
review/fall-2008/american-diplomacy-and-the-foreign-language-challenge

WHO.int. (2005). International Health Regulations (2005). Retrieved from
https://apps.who.int/iris/bitstream/handle/10665/246107/9789241580496-eng.pdf

WHO.int. (2010). A Conceptual Framework for Action on the Social Determinants of
Health. Retrieved from
https://apps.who.int/iris/bitstream/handle/10665/44489/9789241500852_eng.pdf?se
quence=1

WHO.int. (2014-a). Health in All Policies. Retrieved from
https://apps.who.int/iris/bitstream/handle/10665/112636/9789241506908_eng.pdf;j
sessionid=5A3099456028840A395EAFCC1049F7C0?sequence=1

WHO.int. (2014-b). Who statement on the meeting of the International Health
Regulations Emergency Committee concerning the international spread of Wild
Poliovirus. Retrieved from https://www.who.int/news/item/05-05-2014-who-
statement-on-the-meeting-of-the-international-health-regulations-emergency-
committee-concerning-the-international-spread-of-wild-poliovirus

WHO.int. (2018-a). Health equity. Retrieved from https://www.who.int/health-
topics/health-equity#tab=tab_2

WHO.int. (2018-b). Health equity. Retrieved from https://www.who.int/health-
topics/health-equity#tab=tab_1

WHO.int. (2018-c). Health equity. Retrieved from https://www.who.int/health-
topics/health-equity#tab=tab_1

WHO.int. (2018-d). Health inequities and their causes. Retrieved from
https://www.who.int/news-room/facts-in-pictures/detail/health-inequities-and-their-
causes#:~:text=Health%20inequities%20are%20differences%20in,right%20mix%2
0of%20government%20policies.

WHO.int. (2018-e). Health in All Policies as part of the primary health care agenda on
multisectoral action. Retrieved from
https://apps.who.int/iris/bitstream/handle/10665/43541/9241547073_eng.pdf?seque
nce=1&=&isAllowed=y

WHO.int. (2019). Emergencies: International health regulations and emergency
committees. Retrieved from https://www.who.int/news-room/questions-and-
answers/item/emergencies-international-health-regulations-and-emergency-
committees

WHO.int. (2020-a). Who global health and peace initiative (GHPI). Retrieved from
https://www.who.int/initiatives/who-health-and-peace-initiative

WHO.int. (2020-b). WHO-ASPHER Competency Framework for the Public Health
Workforce in the European Region. Retrieved from
https://apps.who.int/iris/bitstream/handle/10665/347866/WHO-EURO-2020-3997-
43756-61569-eng.pdf?sequence=1

WHO.int. (2021-a). Health workforce. Retrieved from
https://www.who.int/data/gho/data/themes/health-workforce

WHO.int. (2021-b). New WHO course strengthens health diplomacy for the pandemic era in the Eastern Mediterranean Region. Retrieved from https://www.emro.who.int/fr/media/actualites/new-who-course-strengthens-health-diplomacy-for-the-pandemic-era-in-the-eastern-mediterranean-region.html

WHO.int. (2022-a). Global Health Needs Global Health Diplomacy. Retrieved from https://www.emro.who.int/health-topics/health-diplomacy/about-health-diplomacy.html

WHO.int. (2022-b). Pandemic influenza preparedness (PIP) framework. Retrieved from https://www.who.int/initiatives/pandemic-influenza-preparedness-framework

WHO.int. (2022-c). Proposed amendments to the international ... Retrieved from https://apps.who.int/gb/wgihr/pdf_files/wgihr2/A_WGIHR2_6-en.pdf

WHO.int. (2022-d). Third round of the global pulse survey on continuity of essential health services during the COVID-19 pandemic. Retrieved from https://www.who.int/publications-detail-redirect/WHO-2019-nCoV-EHS_continuity-survey-2022.1

WHO.int. (2022-e). 14.9 million excess deaths associated with the COVID-19 pandemic in 2020 and 2021. Retrieved from https://www.who.int/news/item/05-05-2022-14.9-million-excess-deaths-were-associated-with-the-COVID-19-pandemic-in-2020-and-2021

WHO.int. (2022-f). New Fund for Pandemic Prevention, Preparedness and response formally established. Retrieved from https://www.who.int/news/item/09-09-2022-new-fund-for-pandemic-prevention--preparedness-and-response-formally-established

WHO.int. (2022-g). Joint external evaluation tool: International Health Regulations (2005) - third edition. Retrieved from https://www.who.int/publications/i/item/9789240051980

WHO.int. (2022-h). Seventy-fifth World Health Assembly to focus on "Health for peace, peace for health" for recovery and Renewal. Retrieved from https://www.who.int/news/item/17-05-2022-seventy-fifth-world-health-assembly-to-focus-on--health-for-peace--peace-for-health--for-recovery-and-renewal

WHO.int. (2023-a). Public health milestones through the years. Retrieved from https://www.who.int/campaigns/75-years-of-improving-public-health/milestones#year-1945

WHO.int. (2023-b). WHO COVID-19 dashboard. Retrieved from
https://COVID19.who.int/

WHO.int. (2023-c). Weekly epidemiological update on COVID-19 - 25 August 2023.
Retrieved from https://www.who.int/publications/m/item/weekly-epidemiological-
update-on-COVID-19---30-august-2023

WHO.int. (2023-d). WHO's Executive Board adopts resolution on access for life-saving
aid into Gaza and respect for laws of war. Retrieved from
https://www.who.int/news/item/10-12-2023-who-s-executive-board-adopts-
resolution-on-access-for-life-saving-aid-into-gaza-and-respect-for-laws-of-war

WHO.int. (2023-e). Pandemic prevention, preparedness and response accord. Retrieved
from https://www.who.int/news-room/questions-and-answers/item/pandemic-
prevention--preparedness-and-response-accord

WHO.int. (2023-f). Governments continue discussions on pandemic agreement
negotiating text. Retrieved from https://www.who.int/news/item/07-12-2023-
governments-continue-discussions-on-pandemic-agreement-negotiating-
text#:~:text=Governments%20lead%20the%20discussions%20on,not%20participat
e%20in%20decision%2Dmaking.

WHO.int. (n.d.-a). Understanding global health through data collection. Retrieved from
https://www.who.int/activities/understanding-global-health-through-data-collection

WHO.int. (n.d.-b). Global Health Ethics. Retrieved from https://www.who.int/health-
topics/ethics-and-health#tab=tab_1

WHO.int. (n.d.-c). Background - International Health Regulations. Retrieved from
https://www.emro.who.int/international-health-regulations/about/background.html

WHO.int. (n.d.-d). International Health Regulations. Retrieved from
https://www.who.int/health-topics/int.ernational-health-regulations#tab=tab_3

WHO.int. (n.d.-e). Global Health Needs Global Health Diplomacy. Retrieved from
https://www.emro.who.int/health-topics/health-diplomacy/about-health-
diplomacy.html

WHO.int. (n.d.-f). Health Diplomacy. Retrieved from https://www.emro.who.int/health-
topics/health-diplomacy/index.html

WHO.int. (n.d.-g). International Health Regulations. Retrieved from
https://www.who.int/health-topics/international-health-regulations#tab=tab_1

WHO.int. (n.d.-h). Assessment of essential public health functions. Retrieved from
https://www.emro.who.int/about-who/public-health-functions/index.html

Williams, B. A., Jones, C. H., Welch, V., & True, J. M. (2023). Outlook of pandemic
preparedness in a post-COVID-19 World. *Nature: NPJ Vaccines, 8*(1).
doi:10.1038/s41541-023-00773-0

Wilson, L., Callender, B., Hall, T. L., Jogerst, K., Torres, H., & Velji, A. (2014).
Identifying Global Health Competencies to Prepare 21st Century Global Health
Professionals: Report from the Global Health Competency Subcommittee of the
Consortium of Universities for Global Health. *Journal of Law, Medicine & Ethics,
42*(S2), 26–31.

Wise, J. (2023). COVID-19: Who declares end of global health emergency. *BMJ.*
doi:10.1136/bmj.p1041

Wiysonge, C. S., Ndwandwe, D., Ryan, J., Jaca, A., Batouré, O., Anya, B.-P. M., &
Cooper, S. (2021). Vaccine hesitancy in the era of COVID-19: Could lessons from
the past help in divining the future? *Human Vaccines & Immunotherapeutics,
18*(1), 1–3. doi:10.1080/21645515.2021.1893062

Wolf, M. (2015). Is there really such a thing as "one health"? thinking about a more than
human world from the perspective of cultural anthropology. *Social Science &
Medicine, 129*, 5–11. doi:10.1016/j.socscimed.2014.06.018

World Bank Group. (2017). From Panic and Neglect to Investing in Health Security:
Financing Pandemic Preparedness at a National Level. Retrieved from
https://www.worldbank.org/en/topic/pandemics/publication/from-panic-neglect-to-
investing-in-health-security-financing-pandemic-preparedness-at-a-national-level

World Bank Group. (2022). Poverty and Shared Prosperity 2022: Correcting Course.
Retrieved from
https://openknowledge.worldbank.org/server/api/core/bitstreams/b96b361a-a806-
5567-8e8a-b14392e11fa0/content

World Bank Group. (2023-a). Chapter 1. *The economic impacts of the COVID-19 crisis.*
Retrieved from https://www.worldbank.org/en/publication/wdr2022/brief/chapter-
1-introduction-the-economic-impacts-of-the-COVID-19-crisis

World Bank Group. (2023-b). Prevent the next pandemic with a one health approach. Retrieved from https://www.worldbank.org/en/news/press-release/2022/10/24/prevent-rather-than-fight-the-next-pandemic-with-a-one-health-approach-world-bank

Worldometer. (2024). Corona virus statistics. Retrieved from https://www.worldometers.info/coronavirus/#countries

Wright, S. (2020). What competencies will leaders need in a new COVID-19 world? *Assessment and Development Matters, 12*(3), 3–6.

Yan, Y., & Saguine, K. (2021). Why we must reimagine capacity building to strengthen education after COVID-19. Retrieved from https://www.weforum.org/agenda/2021/03/why-we-must-reimagine-capacity-building-to-reimagine-education-after-COVID-19/

Zapata, T., Buchan, J., & AzzopardiMuscat, N. (2021). The health workforce: Central to an effective response to the COVID19 pandemic in the European Region. *The International Journal of Health Planning and Management, 36*(S1), 9–13.

Zartman, I. W., & Berman, M. R. (1982). *The Practical Negotiator*. In The Practical Negotiator (pp. 16–27). New Haven u.a.: Yale Univ. Pr.

Zemmel, D. J., Kulik, P. K. G., Leider, J. P., & Power, L. E. (9 2022). Public Health Workforce Development During and Beyond the COVID-19 Pandemic: Findings From a Qualitative Training Needs Assessment. *Journal of Public Health Management and Practice, 28*(Supplement 5), S263–S270.

Zhou, Y. R. (2024). HIV/AIDS, SARS, and COVID-19: The trajectory of China's pandemic responses and its changing politics in a contested World. *Globalization and Health, 20*(1). doi:10.1186/s12992-023-01011-x

Appendices

Appendix 1: Institutional Review Board Exemption:

THE GEORGE WASHINGTON UNIVERSITY

WASHINGTON, DC

Date: November 14, 2023
To: McDonnell, Karen A, PhD
From: The George Washington University Committee on Human Research,
      Institutional Review Board (IRB), FWA00005945
  Subject: IRB# NCR235277 , *"Defining Global Health Diplomacy (GHD) in a Post*
COVID Era: Investigating the knowledge, skills, and core competencies required by
GHD actors to address current and future global health threats."

Exempt Determination Date: 11/14/2023

The request for an exemption determination for the above-referenced study has been completed. The study was determined to be research that is **exempt** from IRB review under DHHS regulatory **category 2**. The project as described in the application may proceed without further oversight by the OHR.

The exemption determination applies only to the project described in your IRB Application. Any changes that may alter in any way the risks to participants, type of information to be accessed, addition of new populations, or change in PI may not be instituted without submission of a Modification within the iRIS system and further review by the OHR prior to implementation of the changes. Please note, it is the responsibility of the GW research team to ensure all approved research personnel have up-to-date CITI training at all times in order to conduct human subjects/participants research.

For Exempt studies involving collaboration with external institutions/sites: Research studies that are registered as exempt are not eligible for institutional reliance agreements. Please reach out to any collaborating site(s) that will be engaged in human subjects research activities on this study to discuss next steps according to their reviewing Institutional Review Board's policies and procedures. If you have questions, please contact the GW Office of Human Research.
Questions or concerns regarding the exemption determination made for the study should be directed to the GW Office of Human Research at ohrirb@gwu.edu or (202) 994-2715.

Appendix 2: Email Interview Request:

Dear [Participant Name]

I hope this email finds you well.

My name is Floramae Esapebong-Ray. I am a third-year DrPH student at George Washington University School of Public Health (Cohort 2021). I am working with Dr. Rebecca Katz on my book topic, "Defining Global Health Diplomacy (GHD) in a post-COVID Era."

I seek to understand the knowledge, skills, and core competencies that Global Health Diplomacy Actors require to practice GHD in a post-COVID era. I would be grateful if you could spare 45 – 60 minutes to participate in a virtual interview at your earliest convenience.

I would love to learn about your perspectives and personal experiences practicing GHD during the recent pandemic and what you think are the necessary knowledge, skills, and core competencies.

I have attached the interview consent form and an information leaflet to provide information about this topic and the scope of the interview questions. Please review both and feel free to ask any questions you may have.

This interview is exploratory, and your responses will be confidential and anonymized by removing any identifying factors such as names, work locations, or affiliate organizations.

Please let me know when you might be available for an interview, and I will send out a Zoom meeting invite. I understand you may have a full-time work schedule, and I will gladly schedule the interview in the evening to accommodate your availability.

Kind regards,

Floramae

Research Topic: Defining Global Health Diplomacy in a post-COVID era
Method: Semi-structured qualitative interviews
Sample Population: US Global Health Diplomacy Actors [Core, Multistakeholder, Informal]
Principal Investigator: Floramae Esapebong-Ray [floramae@gwu.edu | 202-440-3201]
book Committee: Dr. Karen McDonnell (Chair), Dr. Rebecca Katz, Dr. Khadidiatou Ndiaye

Script: Hello, it's lovely to see you! How are you doing today? Thank you for agreeing to speak with me and signing the interview consent form. Although this interview will be recorded, your identity will remain confidential, and any personal identifiers will be excluded from the interview transcript. All data collected will be used solely for the purpose of research and will be securely stored.

This interview will focus on the knowledge, skills, and competencies that Global Health Diplomacy actors need to practice Global Health Diplomacy in a post-COVID era. The study findings will inform the development of Georgetown University's Health Diplomacy Training Initiative to build the capacity of formal and informal GHD actors, making them more fit for the practice of Global Health Diplomacy in a post-COVID era.

A. Skills and core competencies required for Global Health Diplomacy practice

1. To start us off, could you please tell me what skills you think GHD actors need to practice Global Health Diplomacy in a post-COVID era? (Probe: Considering the likelihood of another pandemic like COVID occurring within our lifetime, what skills do you think Global Health Diplomacy would need?)

   Skills are specific learned abilities required to practice Global Health Diplomacy successfully.

2. What core competencies do you think GHD actors need to practice Global Health Diplomacy in a post-COVID era?

   Competencies are the essential knowledge, skills, and abilities that GHD actors need to practice Global Health Diplomacy and properly apply these knowledge, skills, and abilities by GHD actors at the right place and time to practice Global Health Diplomacy effectively.

B. Identifying technical knowledge gaps amongst Global Health Diplomacy actors.

3. What technical knowledge gaps did you face while practicing Global Health Diplomacy during the COVID-19 pandemic? (Probe: What technical knowledge

gaps do you think other Global Health Diplomacy faced while practicing Global
Health Diplomacy during the COVID-19 pandemic?)
Technical knowledge is the practical or theoretical understanding of Global Health
Diplomacy.

Defining Global Health Diplomacy in a post-COVID era

4. Based on the knowledge, skills, and competencies required for practice in a post-
   COVID era. How would you define Global Health Diplomacy in a post-COVID
   era? (Probe: What would you say are the essential qualities and scope of Global
   Health Diplomacy based on the understanding of knowledge, skills, and
   competencies required for practice in a post-COVID era?)

Closing: Thank you again for sharing your experience and insights on this research
project.

5. Is there anything else regarding this you would like to add?
6. Is there anyone in the field of Global Health Diplomacy within the US that you
   could refer me to?

May I contact you again if I have follow-up questions or need further clarification?

Study concept	Definition
Global Health Diplomacy Actors	Individuals, government agencies, institutions, organizations, or entities that cultivate interactions and negotiations between and among each other and within and across governments and states, with the principal objective of improving population health.
Technical knowledge	The practical or theoretical understanding of Global Health Diplomacy.
Skills	Specific learned abilities required to practice Global Health Diplomacy successfully.
Core Competencies	The essential knowledge, skills, and abilities that GHD actors need to practice Global Health Diplomacy and the proper application of these knowledge, skills, and abilities by GHD actors at the right place and time to practice Global Health Diplomacy effectively.
Practice	The real-world application and implementation of Global Health Diplomacy core competencies (knowledge, skills, and abilities) to successfully address global health challenges and achieve global health-related goals.
Define	Describe or explain the meaning of Global Health Diplomacy based on the GHD actor's understanding of knowledge, skills, and competencies required for practice in a post-COVID era.

Appendix 4: Informed Consent Documentation:

Informed Consent Form

Research project title: Defining Global Health Diplomacy in a Post-COVID Era: Investigating the knowledge, skills, and core competencies needed by Global Health Diplomacy Actors

Student Researcher: Floramae Esapebong-Ray

Research Participant's name:

Thank you for agreeing to be interviewed as part of the above research project. Ethical procedures for academic research undertaken from The George Washington University (GWU) require that interviewees explicitly agree to being interviewed and how the information contained in their interview will be used.

The purpose of this research is to understand the knowledge, skills, and core competencies that Global Health Diplomacy Actors require to practice GHD in a post-COVID era. The interview will take 45 minutes without exceeding one hour. We do not anticipate that there are any risks associated with your participation, however, you have the right to stop the interview or withdraw from the research at any time.

This consent form is necessary for us to ensure that you understand the purpose of your involvement and that you agree to the conditions of your participation.

To ensure anonymity your signature is not required, unless you prefer to sign it. If you do not sign the form, your willingness to participate in this research study will be implied if you proceed with research participation. Please keep a copy of this document in case you want to read it again.

Would you therefore read the accompanying information sheet and then sign this form to certify that you approve the following:

1. The interview audio will be recorded through the Zoom platform with automatic transcript generation. The Audio recordings and transcripts will be made available via Zoom at the end of the interview and will hosted on the GWU's password-protected Zoom cloud-based server;
2. The transcript of the interview will be analyzed by Floramae Esapebong-Ray, as research investigator and academic colleagues and researchers with whom she might collaborate as part of the research process;
3. Access to the interview transcript will be limited to the student researcher (Floramae Esapebong-Ray) and academic colleagues and researchers with whom she might collaborate as part of the research process;
4. Any summary interview content, or direct quotations from the interview, that are made available through academic publication or other academic outlets will be anonymized so that you cannot be identified, and care will be taken to ensure that other information in the interview that could identify yourself is not revealed.
5. The actual recording and transcripts will be kept for up to one year after completion of the study and will be deleted from the cloud-based server. The recording will be used solely for data analysis and not for presentation purposes.

Quotation Agreement

All or part of the content of your interview may be used; With regards to being quoted, please initial next to any of the statements that you agree with:

	I also understand that my words may be quoted directly.
	I agree to be quoted directly.
	I agree to be quoted directly if my name is not published and a made-up name (pseudonym) is used.
	I agree that the researchers may publish documents that contain quotations by me.
	I agree that the recording will be used solely for data analysis and not for presentation purposes.

By signing this form I agree that;

1. I am voluntarily taking part in this project. I understand that I don't have to take part, and I can stop the interview at any time;
2. The transcribed interview or extracts from it may be used as described above;
3. I have read the Information sheet;
4. I don't expect to receive any benefit or payment for my participation;
5. I have been able to ask any questions I might have, and I understand that I am free to contact the researcher with any questions I may have in the future.

____

Printed Name

_______________________________________   ___________________

Participants Signature   Date

_______________________________________   ___________________

Researcher's Signature   Date

Contact Information

This research has been reviewed and approved by the George Washington University's Office of Human Research. If you have any further questions or concerns about this study, please contact:

Name of Student Researcher: Floramae Esapebong-Ray
Tel: +1-202-440-3201 | **E-mail:** floramae@gwu.edu

You can also contact Floramae Esapebong-Ray's Research Supervisor

Name of Research Supervisor: Dr. Karen McDonnell | **E-mail:** kmcdonne@gwu.edu

What if I have concerns about this research?

If you are worried about this research, or if you are concerned about how it is being conducted,
you can contact:
The George Washington University Office of Human Research (OHR)
E-mail: ohrirb@gwu.edu
Telephone: 202-994-2715

Appendix 5: Research Study Information Leaflet:

Research Topic: Defining Global Health Diplomacy in a Post-COVID Era
Data Collection Timeline: December 2023 – mid-January 2024
Method: Semi-structured interviews via Zoom
Topic: Defining Global Health Diplomacy in a Post-COVID Era
Target Audience: US Global Health Diplomacy Actors
Student Researcher: Floramae Esapebong-Ray (floramae@gwu.edu | +1- 202-440-3201
Principal Investigator: Karen McDonnell kmcdonne@gwu.edu | Dr. Rebecca Katz
rk952@georgetown.edu

Hello! My name is Floramae Esapebong-Ray. I am a third-year DrPH student at George
Washington University. I am currently working with Dr. Rebecca Katz on my book
topic, "Defining Global Health Diplomacy (GHD) in a post-COVID Era."

I seek to understand the knowledge, skills, and core competencies that Global
Health Diplomacy Actors require to practice GHD in a post-COVID era. I would be
grateful if you could spare 45 – 60 minutes to participate in a virtual interview.
Strengthening Global Health Diplomacy requires GHD actors to have the proper
knowledge, skills, and core competencies to prepare for, prevent, and respond to current
and future global health threats.

I would love to learn about your perspectives and personal experiences practicing
GHD during the recent pandemic and what you think are the necessary knowledge, skills,
and core competencies. This interview is exploratory, and your responses will be
confidential and anonymized by removing any identifying factors such as names, work
locations, or affiliate organizations.

The table below portrays how I will be operationalizing the study concepts within
the research aims and research questions:

Study concept	Definition
Global Health Diplomacy Actors	Individuals, government agencies, institutions, organizations, or entities that cultivate interactions and negotiations between and among each other and within and across governments and states, with the principal objective of improving population health.
Technical knowledge	The practical or theoretical understanding of Global Health Diplomacy
Skills	Specific learned abilities required to successfully practice Global Health Diplomacy

Core Competencies	The essential skills, knowledge, and abilities that GHD actors need to practice Global Health Diplomacy successfully.
Practice	The real-world application and implementation of Global Health Diplomacy core competencies (knowledge, skills, and abilities) to successfully address global health challenges and achieve global health-related goals.
Define	Delineate (identify) the essential qualities and scope of Global Health Diplomacy based on the understanding of knowledge, skills, and competencies required for practice in a post-COVID era.

The study findings will inform the development of Georgetown University's Health Diplomacy Training Initiative to build the capacity of formal and informal GHD actors, making them more fit for the practice of Global Health Diplomacy in a post-COVID era.

The study results will be shared with all the members of the research team, presented publicly during my book defense, and may be published on open-source platforms.

While I cannot offer any participation incentives, your input is invaluable and will contribute to redefining and potentially shaping the field of Global Health Diplomacy.

Please let me know if you have any follow-up questions or concerns about the study, and I look forward to speaking with you.

Kind regards,

Floramae

Appendix 6: Global Health Diplomacy Definitions

Global Health Diplomacy Definitions by Core GHD Actors:

"Global health diplomacy, I would say, is probably twofold; one is actually seeing health as a global issue, which means that you inherently have to deal with this whole complex world of multilateral systems, organizations, economies, trade, all these other global currents that affect health as a global issue. The other way of looking at Global Health Diplomacy is looking at those health problems that truly are global on a massive scale. They might be unique in individual or national applications, but everyone's dealing with them. Or you can look at those health issues which are impacted by global institutions, global trends, global problems" (CORE 6).

"If you're a scientist and all your peers are scientists from all over the world, you have to collaborate and understand the multicultural environment in which you are to be able to produce as a team. Those are people are gonna go back to their countries, and you're gonna have links with them forever. And that's also part of Global Health Diplomacy. The diplomacy comes from your area of [technical] expertise; then, you need skills to be able to interact with the host country. Global Health Diplomacy first has to focus on having a gallery of global health experts that we're sending around the world to represent the best global health interests of the United States. I don't think that Global Health Diplomacy is a thing by itself. It's a lot of effort to expand those links to living in a safer, healthier world, but then diplomacy comes along" (CORE 4).

"Health is hope. People need to be able to wake up in the morning and have hope, and part of that is having good health and knowing that they have a social safety net that'll take care of them if something happens. COVID reminded us that health is also economic capacity. What Health Diplomacy does is have that in the back of the mind that you have some people who want to be buried in their labs or who are doing really important grassroots-level health, because every time they interact with somebody in a clinic, they're saying, 'look, it's a safe place; come here, we will take care of you.' Health is safe. In a post-COVID world, Global Health Diplomacy also recognizes that you cannot only have health people at the table, you have to have these other competencies. You need lawyers, industry people, people in business who are innovative, educators, security people, writers, and yes, you absolutely need health people. If you don't have all of those people at the table, you are not making decisions based on the best available knowledge because we've learned with COVID, with HIV, that an epidemic hits people in their pocket, so it hits all sectors" (CORE 5).

"Global Health Diplomacy is using diplomatic capacities and assets to advance public health goals and looking at health as an opportunity to improve and advance bilateral and multilateral relations. What our Bureau [GHSD] especially wants to do is to have embassies and diplomatic people recognize that health is

always on the agenda. It's not just something that is a response to outbreaks, but that health is one topic in which we can advance bilateral cooperation and understanding, find areas of agreement, and where we want to reduce areas of conflict and disagreement" (CORE 1).

"Global Health Diplomacy is a subset of our diplomatic engagement, and it's one that does require an array of skills for understanding development needs as well as scientific and technical and risk assessment. The ability to work with countries even when we have significant diplomatic differences with them" (CORE 3).

"Global Health Diplomacy is the appropriate application of knowledge and skills to build competence around the practice of Health Diplomacy, meaning advancing your nation's health interests while finding areas of intersection and exploiting them with other nations. And that requires both skills in global health to understand where the areas of intersection are and then diplomacy; understanding in the world of foreign affairs and global governance, how a system would work to advance those interests" (CORE 2).

Global Health Diplomacy Definitions by Multistakeholder GHD Actors:

"Global Health Diplomacy is everywhere because public health is everywhere, and it's everything that we do. By doing this [GHD] and doing it well, we are being proactive and not reactive. It's having a mindset that the threats to public health are international, going past barriers and borders" (MSTK 2).

"Global Health Diplomacy emerged from the fact that health sometimes became an opportunity for better diplomacy, a necessity at the time of pandemics. But I don't prescribe 'in a time of a pandemic or in a time of no pandemic' because there isn't such a thing. I would define Global Health Diplomacy as an emerging area where foreign policy and public health meet at different places to try to bring some coordination in a very messy, uncoordinated world. That's why I said some coordination, being realistic, just because of the very complex world we live in, you cannot just achieve everything" (MSTK 6).

"Global Health Diplomacy is really about ensuring that you, as whichever nation you're representing, are advocating for the health of the population, but also considering that aiding that population is going to contribute to overall global health security and domestic health security. Disease travels very fast via planes, etc., and people move around quickly. So, it's really important that we're providing support to partner governments in a way that respects their sovereignty but also doing it in a way that we're safeguarding the health of our population through those investments. I think it's also about working as an international community in how we aid countries and doing things in a coordinated way with other stakeholders to maximize investments toward improving the health of that country and that community. I think it's also about getting down to the community level at this point rather than nationally. We need to do a better job at engaging local stakeholders because, in the end, these infectious diseases are identified at

the local level and at the health facility. So, if we can equip people there to identify diseases early and report them into the right systems" (MSTK 3).

"Global Health Diplomacy is building trusted relationships and keeping science and evidence at the front, so that we do things and base our decisions and our actions on science and on data, but also ensuring that we don't work in silos, that we work across our partners, across countries, across disciplines, across ministries. So that very, very collaborative openness is really essential. I think we learned that the hard way." (MSTK 7).

"Global Health Diplomacy is a relationship between partners that is underpinned by solving health problems through technical collaborations that one group can bring to the other. But it is also a bidirectional learning exercise: Health Diplomacy is well-executed when you first and foremost connect as human beings. Health diplomacy is evolving, and you should be able to ask those questions and say, 'What do you need help with?' Just because that happens to be my expertise doesn't necessarily mean that that's what is most necessary" (MSTK 1).

"The global health part is health that relates to international matters, not just here in the United States, and diplomacy denotes to me the kind of exchange and barter of ideas and trying to leverage existing partnerships. To put it all together, Global Health Diplomacy, in my definition, would be leveraging partnerships in healthcare globally, beyond the borders of the United States of America into international countries" (MSTK 4).

Global Health Diplomacy Definitions by Informal GHD Actors:

"Global Health Diplomacy is the discipline and skills needed to improve the well-being of people on the planet because it doesn't matter you where you apply that. I didn't say health, because as a physician when we focus on or use the health word, we get stuck in a biomedical definition. And yet you and I know that a lot of the inputs in human well-being have nothing to do with big 'H' Health. Nothing can improve or damage the well-being of people faster than bad political decisions. If I were to use it as a diagram, on one side, we have those technical, medical, and biomedical discoveries that are made; in the middle are the Global Health actors or those with Global Health Diplomacy skills that are essential to be able to bridge that gap between the production of those technical advances, and the people on the other side of that bridge who need them. Global Health Diplomacy is the bridge between discovery and implementation" (INFML 5).

"Regarding a definition of Global Health Diplomacy, I'm not necessarily being crystal clear because I think the attempt to define Global Health Diplomacy or even health diplomacy got so far away from the basic reality. Diplomats do what foreign policymakers tell them to do. It gets really no more complicated than that, and I never really understood the need to build in all these other pieces… Particularly post-COVID, now that we're in a geopolitical world, even more question marks are raised about that. And I certainly don't see any of those actors

from the diplomacy of authoritarian governments, and authoritarianism is on the rise around the world" (INFML 2).

"In a post-COVID era, it's understanding that there's always going to be future outbreak and these skills need to be continuously sharpened. So, it's incumbent on all those who are focused on Global Health Diplomacy to continuously educate themselves on these competencies and continue to build on that skill set. You can't just relax 'cause you never know. Especially on quantitative skills, if you learned that you weren't really good at doing data analysis, then continue to work on that" (INFML 7).

"I look at everybody as potentially being a Global Health Diplomat based on how they would employ diplomacy. And it's beyond just the negotiation skills; it's beyond just learning to be nice because you can't always be nice" (INFML 1).

"I am very much 'global health is local health,' and so every person who works in public health, to me, is a Global Health Diplomat because they could have some interactions in this post-COVID world, considering how virtual we are, with another public health practitioner in another area, and have conversations about lessons learned or sharing best practices. However, I don't necessarily consider a local health department, a global health entity, or a Global Health Diplomacy entity, those are federal" (INFML 4).

"Global Health Diplomacy is engaging in a positive way with counterparts, whether it's organizational counterparts or country or regional counterparts, or stakeholders, and understanding their needs, listening to their needs, understanding the context, and then being able to coordinate, collaborate, and communicate with other stakeholders in order to attend to some of the needs and capacities that the countries or an organization might want to try and develop in-country for dealing with a future pandemic" (INFML 6).